ATTACHMENT THEORY IN CLINICAL WORK WITH CHILDREN

Attachment Theory in Clinical Work with Children

Bridging the Gap between Research and Practice

Edited by

David Oppenheim

Douglas F. Goldsmith

THE GUILFORD PRESS
New York   London

To Anat, Dor, Nadav, and Tamar
—D. O.

To Denise, Joshua, and Elizabeth
—D. F. G.

© 2007 The Guilford Press
A Division of Guilford Publications, Inc.
72 Spring Street, New York, NY 10012
www.guilford.com

Printed in the United States of America

This book is printed on acid-free paper.

Last digit is print number: 9   8   7   6   5   4   3   2   1

Library of Congress Cataloging-in-Publication Data

Attachment theory in clinical work with children : bridging the gap
between research and practice / edited by David Oppenheim, Douglas F.
Goldsmith.
    p. ; cm.
Includes bibliographical references and index.
ISBN-13: 978-1-59385-448-5 (hardcover : alk. paper)
ISBN-10: 1-59385-448-X (hardcover : alk. paper)
    1. Attachment behavior in children.   2. Attachment disorder in
children.   3. Child psychotherapy.   4. Parent and child.   I. Oppenheim,
David, 1958–   II. Goldsmith, Douglas F.
    [DNLM: 1. Object Attachment.   2. Parent–Child
Relations.   3. Child.   WS 105.5.F2 A8836 2007]
    RJ507.A77A93 2007
    618.92′8588—dc22

                                                                    2006037395

About the Editors

David Oppenheim, PhD, is Associate Professor of Psychology at the University of Haifa, Israel, and Associate Editor of *Infant Mental Health Journal.* He has been involved with attachment research for more than 20 years, focusing on the importance of secure, emotionally open parent–child relations for children's development and mental health. Dr. Oppenheim has also studied how secure attachments are fostered by parental insightfulness into the child's inner world, and has applied attachment concepts and methods in research on clinical populations. He is actively involved in lecturing and writing on the clinical applications of attachment.

Douglas F. Goldsmith, PhD, is a practicing psychologist and Executive Director of The Children's Center, in Salt Lake City, Utah, which specializes in the treatment of families with infants, toddlers, and preschoolers. His work focuses on the assessment and treatment of attachment problems, and he has published several articles regarding the application of attachment theory to clinical practice. Dr. Goldsmith holds adjunct faculty appointments in the Departments of Educational Psychology, Psychology, and Psychiatry at the University of Utah.

Contributors

Inga Blom, MA, Department of Psychology, New School University, New York, New York

Amy L. Busch, PhD, Department of Psychiatry, University of California, and Child Trauma Research Project, San Francisco General Hospital, San Francisco, California

Glen Cooper, MA, Marycliff Institute, Spokane, Washington

Debra D'Agostino, MA, Department of Psychology, New School University, New York, New York

Smadar Dolev, PhD, Department of Psychology, University of Haifa, Haifa, Israel

Mary Dozier, PhD, Department of Psychology, University of Delaware, Newark, Delaware

Douglas F. Goldsmith, PhD, The Children's Center, Salt Lake City, Utah

Damion Grasso, MA, Department of Psychology, University of Delaware, Newark, Delaware

Kay Henderson, MSc, Department of Psychology, University College London, and Anna Freud Centre, London, United Kingdom

Saul Hillman, MSc, Department of Psychology, University College London, and Anna Freud Centre, London, United Kingdom

Jill Hodges, PhD, Brain and Behavioral Sciences Unit, Institute of Child Health; Anna Freud Centre; and Child and Adolescent Mental Health Service, Department of Psychological Medicine, Great Ormond Street Hospital for Sick Children, London, United Kingdom

Kent Hoffman, PhD, Marycliff Institute, Spokane, Washington

Jeanne Kaniuk, BA, Coram Family, London, United Kingdom

Nina Koren-Karie, PhD, School of Social Work, University of Haifa, Haifa, Israel

Erin Lewis, BA, Department of Psychology, University of Delaware, Newark, Delaware

Alicia F. Lieberman, PhD, Department of Psychiatry, University of California, and Child Trauma Research Project, San Francisco General Hospital, San Francisco, California

Oliver Lindhiem, BA, Department of Psychology, University of Delaware, Newark, Delaware

Robert Marvin, PhD, The Mary D. Ainsworth Child–Parent Attachment Clinic and Department of Psychology, University of Virginia, Charlottesville, Virginia

David Oppenheim, PhD, Center for the Study of Child Development and Department of Psychology, University of Haifa, Haifa, Israel

Bert Powell, MA, Marycliff Institute, Spokane, Washington

Shahaf Salomon, MA, Department of Psychology, Hebrew University of Jerusalem, Jerusalem, Israel

Efrat Sher-Censor, MA, Department of Psychology, University of Haifa, Haifa, Israel

Arietta Slade, PhD, Yale Child Study Center, Yale University, New Haven, Connecticut

Howard Steele, PhD, Department of Psychology, New School University, New York, New York

Miriam Steele, PhD, Department of Psychology, New School University, New York, New York

Nurit Yirmiya, PhD, Department of Psychology and School of Education, Hebrew University of Jerusalem, Jerusalem, Israel

Charles H. Zeanah, MD, Department of Psychiatry and Neurology, Tulane University Health Sciences Center, New Orleans, Louisiana

Preface

The 1991 biennial meeting of the Society for Research in Child Development (SRCD) in Seattle, Washington, featured a symposium on the clinical applications of attachment theory. Mary Ainsworth, along with Mary Main and additional speakers, addressed a room filled with attentive participants who were eager to learn how to begin to address attachment concerns in clinical practice. The ideas were fascinating but also challenging: While it was clear that advances in attachment theory and research could have tremendous potential value for clinicians, there was also a clear message of caution regarding the complexities and pitfalls of applying research-based theories and methods in the clinical setting. The field was confronted once again with the perennial science–practice gap: High-quality and clinically pertinent knowledge was being accumulated in university laboratories, but this knowledge was not reaching the frontline clinician. This was not only a matter of disseminating research findings. There was the more profound issue of adapting research concepts and methods to clinical work in a way that would maintain their integrity while also being sufficiently flexible and meaningful to meet the complexity of the individual case—be it child, parent, or family.

We were both very familiar with this tension from our everyday work, particularly from our experience teaching attachment theory and research to clinicians. The research papers were filled with information that we felt was extremely valuable and addressed many lacunae in clinical theories, but the leap from these papers to the clinical case was usually left for the reader to venture. The pivotal SRCD symposium and our belief in the clinical value of attachment research spurred us to organize a series of conferences focused on "bridging the gap" between attachment research and clinical application. The conference series, sponsored by the Children's Center in Salt Lake City, Utah, began in 1999 and has been taking place annually since then. We invited leading researchers/clinicians to talk about how they took the research concepts and methods they were developing when "wearing the researcher hat" and applied them clinically when "wearing the clinician hat." This book is a result of this conference series as well as additional meetings where, as a group, we attempted to tackle the issues inherent in the clinical application of a complex theory (see also the special issue of *Infant Mental Health Journal* [Vol. 25, No. 4, July–August 2004] devoted to clinical applications of attachment theory in which prior publications emanating from our group were published). Each chapter lays out original ideas, concepts, and methods that represent the state of the art in attachment research, and the authors describe not only the implications of the research for clinical work but also, using clinical case material, how the attachment perspective is actually applied. In other words, the reader is escorted across the science–practice divide by experienced guides familiar with both territories.

It is of course no coincidence that attachment research has yielded so much clinically relevant knowledge. After all, attachment theory has deep roots in the clinical world. It was developed by John Bowlby with the aim of offering clinicians a powerful and scientifically based theory that would replace outdated notions and guide clinical practice. The theory offered hypotheses regarding the origins of psychopathology in early separation experiences as well as other adverse emotional experiences, particularly those embedded in the parent–child relationship. It also offered many insights regarding the appropriate treatment for such psychopathology. These innovative ideas were not met with much enthusiasm by the clinical community, however. In fact, many of Bowlby's colleagues shunned his theory and saw it as irrelevant for their work. The community of academic psychology, however, showed more openness to attachment theory, particularly after the research of Mary Ainsworth, a clinical and developmental psychologist, supported many of Bowlby's notions. Ainsworth's painstaking observations of early interactions between mothers and their infants provided powerful confirmation of Bowlby's hypotheses regarding the function and significance of early attachments. The acceptance of attachment theory grew even more following the publication of Ainsworth's studies of the Strange Situation procedure, an observational paradigm designed to assess the security of the affectional bond between infant and parent. This observational procedure opened the way to the reliable assessment of individual differences in attachment and helped define and conceptualize the expression of security and anxiety in early relationships. During the 1980s and 1990s attachment theory became increasingly accepted and influential within the field of developmental psychology, to the point that it is considered by many as the most persuasive theory of early emotional development. Moreover, the influence of attachment theory expanded gradually beyond developmental psychology to include social and clinical psychology as well.

Based on its solid grounding in normative research, the interest in clinical applications of attachment theory began to grow around the mid-1980s. A particularly important additional impetus for these applications was the expansion of attachment research into the representational domain. Marked primarily by the development of the Adult Attachment Interview by Mary Main and her colleagues, attachment research was beginning to address not only attachment bonds as behavioral patterns of the child vis-à-vis the parent, but also the evolution of these patterns into representational models in the mind of the developing child. Attachment research was now tackling the issue of how parents' past relationship experiences, as well as the interaction between them and their children, are reflected in meaning structures in the mind of the child—an issue of great interest and relevance for clinical work. These developments as well as additional influences led to a growing number of clinical attachment studies, with researchers using the concepts and methods developed in normative studies in order to address clinical questions and develop attachment-based interventions. Thus, three or four decades after Bowlby's publication of the first volume of his *Attachment* trilogy and the non-acceptance of his ideas by the clinical community, attachment research had returned to addressing clinical issues, and the present volume is part of this body of work. But this book tries to take clinical application one step further. The authors of all chapters were asked not only to conceptually apply attachment ideas and methods to clinical issues. In addition, they share with readers how these concepts and methods can be used in the actual clinical encounter, and they illustrate, using case material, the unique contributions of an attachment perspective.

We envision the main audience for the book as clinicians working with children and their families who are interested in deepening their understanding of the clinical application of attachment concepts and the added value of an attachment perspective for both assessment and intervention. While the chapters all provide theoretical and research background, the book assumes familiarity with the basic concepts and methods of attachment and does not provide an overview of the theory. With the immense advances made in attachment over the past decades, covering the basics of attachment would require a volume in and of itself! Moreover, excellent introductions and reviews of attachment research are available (e.g., Cassidy and Shaver's *Handbook of Attachment* [1999]), and the reader is invited to consult these resources.

The book is also intended for a research audience. Researchers less familiar with the clinical world may find much excitement and satisfaction in the usefulness of research-based methods and ideas for clinicians, and ultimately for the families and children seeking help. In addition, researchers are likely to discover in the pages of this book how clinical applications stretch accepted theories to their limit, expose areas that require additional investigation, and raise new questions for future studies. Bridging the gap between science and practice is not a one-sided effort focused on translating science to practice—it is a two-way street that can benefit the researcher as much as it does the clinician.

OVERVIEW OF THE BOOK

The book is divided into two parts. The first includes five chapters that describe the clinical application of research-based methods, particularly those that focus on assessing various aspects of parenting, and the second includes four chapters that describe psychotherapeutic interventions with children and parents based on attachment principles.

The first chapter, by Charles Zeanah, describes how the author uses an interview designed to assess parents' representations of their children, the Working Model of the Child Interview, as part of the assessment and treatment of a mother–infant dyad presenting with significant relationship difficulties. The chapter provides extended excerpts from the interview, with the clinician's thoughts, observations, and hypotheses presented following the mother's responses. Thus, the reader is provided with an opportunity to "sit on the shoulder" of the clinician and follow the development of his impressions and hypotheses as he uses the interview to better understand the mother's experience of her infant and herself as a mother. The chapter also includes the formulation of the case, how it was shared with the mother, and information about the treatment.

Nina Koren-Karie and colleagues also focus on the representation of the child by the parent, specifically on the capacity for *insightfulness*, that is, seeing the world from the child's point of view. The chapter describes two mothers of preschoolers referred for treatment that involved their children and themselves, and discusses their pre- and posttreatment Insightfulness Assessments. Using examples from the pre- and posttreatment interviews, the chapter illustrates the specific markers of difficulties in insightfulness, and the gains in insightfulness made by both mothers. The chapter also highlights how, even in the noninsightful pretreatment interviews, positive signs forecasting the gains made by these mothers could be detected—information crucial for developing a balanced view of parents who show significant difficulties being empathic to their children and planning therapeutic work with them.

In the next chapter, Miriam Steele and colleagues apply an attachment perspective to the assessment and treatment of maltreated children who were later adopted. The chapter stresses that careful observations of play interactions between parents and their recently adopted children can identify parental "attachment-facilitative behaviors" that are crucial for the development of the attachment relationships of these severely traumatized children. It also describes how reflecting the insights gleaned from these observations back to the parents can help them gain new and more positive perspectives regarding their children, and overcome their natural tendency to withdraw in response to the seemingly rejecting behavior of these children.

In the fourth chapter, Mary Dozier and colleagues discuss the implications of the commitment foster parents feel toward the children they are fostering for the development of these children. The chapter introduces the This Is My Baby interview, designed to assess the thoughts and feelings of foster parents regarding their foster children. Parents' responses in this interview can be used to assess their level of commitment toward the children they foster, and the chapter provides extensive examples of high, medium, and low commitment. The chapter also reports on child and parent characteristics that may explain why some foster parents are more committed than others, and provides an attachment-based theoretical account of why lack of commitment can have such devastating effects on the development of children in foster care.

David Oppenheim and colleagues discuss in the fifth chapter the emotional processes parents go through after they receive a significant developmental diagnosis for their child, and the powerful impact these processes can have for children's development. Using an attachment framework regarding loss and its resolution, the chapter discusses why lack of acceptance and resolution of the child's diagnosis may have adverse implications for the parent–child relationship. Examples from the Reaction to Diagnosis Interview illustrate the expression of resolution in parental interviews, with an emphasis on how both resolution and lack of resolution can be expressed in multiple ways. The chapter also reviews research findings regarding resolution and discusses their implications for clinical work with parents of children who have received a developmental diagnosis.

The second section of the book opens with a chapter by Amy Busch and Alicia Lieberman, who bring together two important lines of research: trauma research, which delineates the harmful impact of traumatic stress on young children, and attachment research, which discusses the importance of secure attachment for moderating the impact of trauma and helping children recover. They stress that a "dual lens" based on attachment and trauma theories is needed for treating young children who have been exposed to trauma. The chapter includes an extensive mother–child case involving two young children who have been exposed to domestic violence and shows how child–parent psychotherapy can be used to disentangle the reciprocal impact of attachment and trauma and return children to a healthier developmental course.

The next chapter, by Bert Powell and colleagues, presents the Circle of Security model, an early intervention program based on attachment theory and research and designed to help caregivers reevaluate their internal representations of the child and the self to match the emotional needs of their children. The intervention is provided in a group format for mothers of young children and makes extensive use of carefully selected and edited video recordings of the child and the mother that are used to enhance maternal reflectiveness. The chapter begins with a review of the intervention model. This is followed by a detailed case that illustrates the implementation of the model, with the authors going back and forth between theory and clinical case material to provide the theoretical rationale for the intervention and to discuss the responses of the mother. The significance of role reversal in parents particularly sensitive to separation is highlighted, as is the therapeutic necessity to help parents experience an "empathic shift" regarding their child's emotional world.

The penultimate chapter, by Douglas Goldsmith, describes a therapeutic preschool program based on attachment principles. The core idea is that the intervention, which combines parent–child work with the therapeutic preschool program, challenges the negative internal working models the young children have formed based on their histories of rejection, maltreatment, and trauma. The chapter explains how these internal working models act as self-fulfilling prophecies and often perpetuate additional negative cycles, even when children encounter new and positive social partners. Next, the chapter describes in detail the strategies used in the preschool in order to challenge children's negative expectations and help them experience peers, therapists, and themselves in a new and more positive light. The relationship focus of the intervention is exemplified using the detailed case of a 2-year-old adopted child and her mother. The case illustrates how the child's negative internal working models underlay her fear, extreme aggression, and desperate need for protection. The case also illustrates how the preschool program helped the child feel safe and rely on others, and how parent–child sessions helped the mother appreciate the emotional needs underlying the child's difficult and rejecting behavior.

The book closes with a chapter by Arietta Slade that illustrates the usefulness of "keeping the child in mind" while doing long-term individual work with adults. Slade introduces the concept of disorganized attachment and presents the theorizing regarding its roots in frightened and/or frightening parental behavior as well as in helpless and/or hostile parental states of mind. Next, hypotheses are presented regarding the implication of such experiences for adults' fragmented awareness of painful mental states involving trauma, and these provide the background for the case presentation. The case illustrates disorganization both at the level of the client's relationships with her parents and in her own caregiving. In addition, these difficulties are played out in the relationship with the therapist, leading her to experience much of the emotional dysregulation, fear, and dissociation experienced by the client. Slade finds attachment theorizing and behavioral descriptions regarding the origins of disorganization particularly useful in helping the therapist imagine the client's experience, put it into words that are experience near, and increase empathy for the fear underlying attempts to seek care.

In closing, we hope the readers of this book will share our excitement about the diverse applications of advances in attachment research for clinical work. It is our belief that these chapters elucidate the usefulness of an attachment approach for enhancing our empathic understanding of children, parents, and individuals seeking help to overcome emotional difficulties and relational barriers rooted in their past and current attachment relationships.

REFERENCE

Cassidy, J., & Shaver, P. R. (Eds.). (1999). *Handbook of attachment: Theory, research, and clinical applications.* New York: Guilford Press.

Contents

PART I. CLINICAL USE OF ATTACHMENT
RESEARCH ASSESSMENTS

ONE   Constructing a Relationship Formulation   3
for Mother and Child: Clinical Application
of the Working Model of the Child Interview
Charles H. Zeanah

TWO   Keeping the Inner World of the Child in Mind: 31
Using the Insightfulness Assessment with Mothers
in a Therapeutic Preschool
Nina Koren-Karie, David Oppenheim,
and Douglas F. Goldsmith

THREE Intervening with Maltreated Children   58
and Their Adoptive Families: Identifying
Attachment-Facilitative Behaviors
Miriam Steele, Jill Hodges, Jeanne Kaniuk,
Howard Steele, Debra D'Agostino, Inga Blom,
Saul Hillman, and Kay Henderson

FOUR   The Role of Caregiver Commitment in Foster Care: 90
        Insights from the This Is My Baby Interview
        Mary Dozier, Damion Grasso, Oliver Lindhiem,
        and Erin Lewis

FIVE   Parental Resolution of the Child's Diagnosis   109
        and the Parent–Child Relationship:
        Insights from the Reaction to Diagnosis Interview
        David Oppenheim, Smadar Dolev, Nina Koren-Karie,
        Efrat Sher-Censor, Nurit Yirmiya,
        and Shahaf Salomon

PART II. ATTACHMENT THEORY AND PSYCHOTHERAPY

SIX   Attachment and Trauma: An Integrated Approach   139
        to Treating Young Children Exposed
        to Family Violence
        Amy L. Busch and Alicia F. Lieberman

SEVEN   The Circle of Security Project: A Case Study—   172
        "It Hurts to Give That Which You Did Not Receive"
        Bert Powell, Glen Cooper, Kent Hoffman,
        and Robert Marvin

EIGHT   Challenging Children's Negative Internal   203
        Working Models: Utilizing Attachment-Based
        Treatment Strategies in a Therapeutic Preschool
        Douglas F. Goldsmith

NINE   Disorganized Mother, Disorganized Child: 226
        The Mentalization of Affective Dysregulation
        and Therapeutic Change
        Arietta Slade

        Index   251

PART I

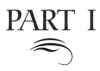

Clinical Use of Attachment
Research Assessments

CHAPTER ONE

Constructing a Relationship Formulation for Mother and Child
Clinical Application of the Working Model of the Child Interview

CHARLES H. ZEANAH

One of the most significant advancements in attachment research occurred when Main, Kaplan, and Cassidy (1985) published their seminal paper on the Adult Attachment Interview (AAI). This paper represented a breakthrough for several reasons. First, it provided a method for assessing parental characteristics that were strongly associated with infant Strange Situation classifications; this had not been achieved previously in any consistent or compelling manner. Second, by focusing on narrative qualities of parents' descriptions of their attachment histories, Main and colleagues (1985) shifted the focus from what parents said to how they said it. Evaluating parents' statements about their infants had long been central to clinical work with infants and families, but the AAI introduced a formal method for assessing specific narrative qualities, an approach that may be usefully applied in clinical settings (Boris, Fueyo,

& Zeanah, 1997). Third, Main and colleagues (1985) specifically linked the construct of what is measured by the AAI to representations, thereby linking it to the findings of cognitive psychology and Bowlby's (1969/ 1982) theorizing about internal working models.

Following this important breakthrough, our group developed the Working Model of the Child Interview (WMCI; Zeanah, Benoit, & Barton, 1986), which was designed to assess a parent's representation of a particular child. It was developed explicitly to be a clinically useful research method. The interview and coding system and their clinical application have been described in detail elsewhere (Zeanah & Benoit, 1995; Zeanah, Larrieu, Valliere, & Heller, 2000), but briefly, it is a semistructured interview that was designed to elicit parents' descriptions of their infants and young children. As with the AAI, from which it was derived, the WMCI includes a formal coding system focused on qualitative features of the narrative, but we have found that the interview is clinically useful even without regard to the coding system.

As a research measure, the WMCI has been validated in a number of published studies (Benoit, Parker, & Zeanah, 1997; Benoit, Zeanah, Parker, Nicholson, & Coolbear, 1997; Huth-Bocks, Levendosky, Bogat, & von Eye, 2004; Huth-Bocks, Levendosky, Theran, & Bogat, 2004; Rosenblum, McDonough, Muzik, Miller, & Sameroff, 2002; Rosenblum, Zeanah, McDonough, & Muzik, 2004; Schechter et al., 2005; Zeanah, Benoit, Hirshberg, Barton, & Regan, 1994). It has been shown to be stable, to be associated with mother and child's interactive behaviors, and to be meaningfully associated with both risk conditions and clinical status.

The purpose of this chapter is to illustrate in detail how use of the WMCI in a clinical setting can contribute to an understanding of a particular infant–parent relationship and provide important indicators as to how treatment might proceed. After introducing the model of relationship assessment that guided the case, I describe the assessment in some detail. Most of the chapter is devoted to excerpts from the WMCI and commentaries about how the material was integrated with other data and used to develop a treatment plan. Following this, I present the formulation derived from the evaluation and summarize the treatment that actually was implemented. The goal is to have the reader witness the construction of a clinical formulation as the material from the interview presents itself. Thus, some of the quotes are more extended than is typical, but the purpose of the quotes is to engage the reader in trying to understand how a particular mother understood and experienced her infant, and to consider how her representation of the child might lead toward or away from certain treatment approaches.

MODEL OF RELATIONSHIP ASSESSMENT

My colleagues and I have elsewhere described an approach to relationship assessment (Zeanah et al., 2000). Briefly, following Stern-Bruschweiler and Stern (1989), we considered both external (observable interactions) and internal (subjective perceptions) components of the infant–parent relationships important to assess. Sometimes interactions are considered synonymous with relationships, but their model makes clear that interactions are only the observable, recurrent patterns of behavior that parents and infants engage in. The parent's subjective experience of who the baby is, or representations of the infant, may be assessed formally, while the infant's subjective experience must be inferred. The case is used to demonstrate how we assessed and integrated these components.

INTRODUCTION TO THE CASE

The case below is of a young infant and his mother whom I believed had a relationship disorder. Because of this, in assessing and later treating the case, I was somewhat less concerned with traditional signs and symptoms in the infant that led to the referral and somewhat more interested in the quality of the mother–infant relationship. This interest led me to try to understand the meaning of the infant's behavior toward his mother and toward me as a primary focus of treatment.

The main themes that were revealed in the course of the WMCI included the mother's self-deprecatory style, her feeling rejected by the baby, her lack of spousal support, and her desire to be a perfect mother, worrying constantly that she was not doing enough. In addition, there was an implicit expectation for the infant to be perfect also and to gratify her neediness and her wish for control. Each of these themes contributed to her experience of who the infant was for her.

The reader will note that the comments become longer and more detailed as the interview progresses. This is because I did not have a formulation initially, but developed one gradually as the interview unfolded and the mother revealed more about herself, the baby, and their relationship. Rather than go back and retrospectively add in detailed components of the formulation, I have chosen instead to allow the reader to learn how the seeds of the formulation took root initially and later grew into my fuller understanding of the case.

INITIAL REFERRAL

An experienced pediatrician called to say that he was referring a 3-month-old infant who was having sleep and feeding difficulties and who had the "most anxious mother" the pediatrician had seen in 15 years of practice.

The baby had been born following an uncomplicated pregnancy to a 35-year-old married, first-time mother. She explained that she had a number of concerns about the baby. She felt that he was excessively irritable, crying on and off all day, and that he seemed to need her constant attention or he became fussy. He also had feeding problems in that he seemed to be hungry every hour, but he refused to nurse for long. He also only nursed on the left breast, and he seemed to prefer a nipple shield to the breast. She said that he had initially "overslept," but more recently he seemed not to sleep more than 1 to 1.5 hours at a time. She also had a number of concerns about whether or not the baby was developing as he should because he did not seem to be engaging the world in the way that she had read that he should. She and the baby, it was clear, were both exhausted.

The mother had sought help from her pediatrician, and she also was a voracious reader of books and magazine articles about parenting and infant development. Although her supports were somewhat limited, she also had received advice from a number of her extended family members and friends about how best to manage the baby. Despite all of this help, problems seemed to be worsening.

The mother was a professional on leave from her job, and her husband of 6 years was a self-employed small businessman. She hinted that her marriage was strained, in part because the hoped-for closeness in her marriage that she felt the baby would bring had not materialized. Her relationships with her own family were strained, and her in-laws lived in another state. All of this left her feeling somewhat isolated and unsupported.

She recalled her father when she was growing up as "distant and aloof" and "hard to please," and her mother as involved but demanding, "angry," and "difficult to satisfy." She had been a high achiever in school, at times her only source of esteem, and she was very proud of her graduate degree.

INTERACTIONAL ASSESSMENT

In a second session, mother and baby were seen in a face-to-face interaction paradigm (Tronick, Als, Adamson, Wise, & Brazelton, 1978), which is designed to optimize conditions for social interaction between young infants and their caregivers. In the version that we used in this case, there were four episodes, each lasting 2 minutes: (1) play/talk with your baby the way you usually do; (2) get the best from the baby that you can; (3) still-face; and (4) play/talk with the baby the way that you usually do.

The interaction was remarkable. Immediately, in close proximity to the baby's face, the mother began staring intently, talking, laughing, and touching the baby in a barrage of stimulation. In response, the baby squirmed, gaze averted, and at times seemed almost to gulp for air. The stimulation continued unabated for the first 4 minutes of the procedure until the still-face episode began. At that point, with the mother making eye contact, the baby began for the first time to look directly into his mother's eyes. Although the still-face episode usually involves some degree of distress or other potent disengagement cues from the baby, in this case, the baby seemed riveted to his mother's face and eyes. He maintained direct eye contact for almost the entire 2-minute episode.

This reaction was just the opposite of what one typically observes. Because the still-face episode includes an unresponsive parent, the baby's expectation for social responsiveness is violated. As a result, most babies become distressed or dysregulated during the still-face episode. This infant, however, seemed better able to "take in" his mother when she was in the still-face episode and not overwhelming him with stimulation.

EXCERPTS FROM THE WORKING MODEL OF THE CHILD INTERVIEW

The interview was administered in a separate session, following the interactional assessment. Although we usually recommend that the parent be alone during the interview, so as not to be distracted, with young infants it is not uncommon for mothers to prefer to keep the baby during the interview. In this case the infant was present during the interview, and some of the mother's and infant's behavior is noted in the excerpts that follow.

Excerpt 1

CLINICIAN: Let's go back to the beginning of the pregnancy and tell me about that. Was it planned, or a surprise?

MOTHER: It was very planned on my part. We had been married 6½ years, 6 years at the time. And I had wanted the baby since the day I got married (*chuckle*), and it never seemed to happen, and then I bought the ovulation predictor test and the thing turned blue, and I told my husband, "It's now or never." I got pregnant the first month that I tried, and um . . .

CLINICIAN: How'd you feel about it?

MOTHER: I was thrilled, but I was scared to death because I, because I am kind of a neurotic person, and I was so afraid I was going to breathe something wrong or eat something wrong or fall and was very, very nervous throughout the whole pregnancy, so I probably didn't enjoy it the way that I should have because I was convinced that something was going to go wrong. And then I had a lot of nausea in the first few months. I guess a lot of women do. And when I threw up, nothing tasted good. And I was trying to shovel broccoli down my throat even though I couldn't stand it. I guess everybody goes through that.

CLINICIAN: How did your husband react?

MOTHER: He was shocked, because he, um, I'd—I had been talking about getting pregnant for 6 years and it never happened and I don't think he really ever really thought . . . I guess he thought that it would happen some day, but never really thought about it as being a reality. And umm, I think he was stunned. And then throughout the pregnancy, I have to say I was disappointed. He wasn't, he was looking forward to the baby, but he wasn't really into the pregnancy. And he would say, "Well, I can't really get into it." I would say, "Won't you read this with me?" or "Won't you look at that?" or "Don't you want to talk about this or that?" And he said, "I can't really get into something that's going to happen 5 months from now." Even when I was pregnant, I don't think it was really a reality to him. And then, I signed us up for the childbirth classes and he really hated going to those and fell asleep during one of them and mortified me. Um, I just don't think . . . he never really wanted to feel the baby you know, which was a disappointment also to me. But when the baby did come during delivery, he was fantastic. I couldn't believe how he just, he was like monitoring my contractions and he was just totally into it. It was wonderful. So that worked out okay even though it was a disappointment during the pregnancy.

Comment: The initial probes on the WMCI are similar to a developmental history, except that the emphasis is less on the facts and the detail about the baby's history and more about the parent's experience of the baby. This emphasis is more telling about the parent's relationship with the baby, as it reflects subjective experience rather than the facts of developmental history. The WMCI, like other attachment interviews, relies in part on narrative qualities. Therefore, the mother's story of the baby is important. What is notable in this initial excerpt is the palpable anxiety and disappointment that the mother had experienced regarding the baby even before he was born. Since these remained important clinical issues at the time of referral, it seemed important that they had been evident, and associated with marital disappointment, even prior to birth. Also striking was her sense of aloneness and lack of support, from her husband and from her own family. Often, such lack of support means that the baby may be looked to provide some of the support that is lacking in other relationships and may be associated with role reversal.

Excerpt 2

CLINICIAN: Let me ask you something else. What sort of impressions did you have about the baby before he was born?

MOTHER: Um, well I had amniocentesis, so I knew that he was going to be a boy. Then, I figured he would be a boy because I didn't want to count my chickens, because I had heard that sometimes it could be wrong, so. Um, what kind of impressions did I have?

CLINICIAN: What sort of personality did you'd think he'd have?

MOTHER: Ah, um (*chuckle*), I thought he'd be a sweet little angel (*laughs, again*).

Comment: Although it is not uncommon for parents' prenatal representations of their infants to be overwhelmingly positive (Zeanah, Zeanah, & Stewart, 1990), the contrast between this mother's prenatal perceptions and her struggle with the baby after birth were notable. It seemed possible that she had idealized the child, sustaining herself through an anxious pregnancy with the reassuring image of a "sweet little angel" who would make it all better for her. My question was, how much out of the normal range was her idealization?

Excerpt 3

MOTHER: I thought that they slept a lot, but then when he did sleep a lot, I worried so much that he was sleeping too much. This, you see, this is how he gives a cry, he just (*makes a crowing noise to demonstrate the baby's cry*). All right, sweetheart (*comforting baby*).

CLINICIAN: Crows a little bit?

MOTHER: Yeah, you want to fly? Want to fly? (*She is trying to quiet the baby by swinging him to and fro in front of her.*) Um, I don't know, you know? I didn't know what to expect. I guess I just expected this little Gerber baby, you know. That would just, um. I didn't think they could do so much so young. To be quite honest, I thought they just kind of were a sleepy thing in your arms for like 6 to 8 months. I just didn't really . . . he didn't look the way that I thought that he would look. He came out with all of this hair and he looks different than what I thought he would look.

CLINICIAN: So there've been some surprises?

MOTHER: Yes.

Comment: This description conveys some of the mother's confusion and bewilderment. Her surprise at his appearance seemed connected at a deeper level to her surprise by many aspects of his behavior and personality that made him not what she expected. This added to the earlier concern that the (over)idealized prenatal image had left her unprepared for the baby she met at delivery. Large discrepancies between prenatal

expectations and postnatal perceptions often reflect relationship disturbances.

Excerpt 4

(*Baby is crying and agitated.*)

MOTHER: He came a month early, and it was a holiday weekend. Oh,
shh, shh, shh (*comforting the baby*). Wouldn't it be nice if we just
ate something? Let's try that. (*Begins to nurse the baby.*) Won't you
try that? No? (*Pulls baby away from her breast.*) Um, my parents
had been down for the holiday and were staying with us and Daniel. All right, all right. (*Stands with the baby and begins swinging
him.*) I could do this for an hour.

CLINICIAN: Is this what you do when he gets upset?

MOTHER: Yes, yes, I do, and I do this until my back breaks, and I can't
stand it anymore.

Comment: Here, several things were notable—though it was the
interaction rather than the narrative that was striking. Up to this point,
the mother had demonstrated a low threshold for responding to fussiness in the baby. Now that the baby was actually crying, it was clear that
she was unable to soothe the baby effectively, despite making remarkable efforts to do so by swinging the baby back and forth, uncomfort-
ably fully extending him in front of her body, illustrating the struggle she
experienced to be a "good" mother. Somehow, this image seemed to capture her struggle to be the kind of mother she wanted to be but also her
feelings of ineffectiveness.

Excerpt 5

CLINICIAN: Tell me about labor and delivery.

MOTHER: I was just a little disappointed for a long time because I, um,
because everything was in so much chaos and because I had, my husband had never really wanted to discuss things. I had really wanted to
breast-feed him on the delivery table and hold him, and everything
was so, I was just so wiped out from delivery that I forgot to breast-
feed him. And I forgot to say that I wanted to hold him, that they just
kind of swept him away from me and took him away. First it was 5

hours, and then they gave him back to me. Then, as soon as they gave him back to me, he spit up, and so they took him away again for another 3 hours. And after that I just felt so disappointed that I didn't have this. I had pictured this beautiful breast-feeding thing on the delivery table. And I just forgot! My brain went right out the window. And, um, and when they did put him in my arms, my husband was off making phone calls to tell people, and I felt that he probably should have been with us and that the phone calls could have waited a while. So that was very disappointing, I have to say, but the delivery itself was a very good experience. I didn't need any medication, and my husband was right there.

Comment: Again, the mother's disappointment in comparing her actual experience to her imagined experience is palpable. Furthermore, both her self-deprecation and her hurt that her husband was not there for her are evident again. These themes were elaborated more fully later in the interview and during treatment.

Excerpt 6

CLINICIAN: I want to see if you can sit.

MOTHER: (*Still standing, swings the baby in her arms.*) OK. Do you want to sit down, little boy? Um, that's a good boy. (*The baby begins to cry loudly as she places him in an infant seat.*) Ah, will you be good little boy? (*Pats the baby's forehead.*) Ah, fussy? I better rock him, or should I leave him there? (*Looks at the clinician befuddled and shrugs her shoulders beseechingly.*)

CLINICIAN: Can you rock him with him sitting there?

MOTHER: I can try. (*Begins to rock the infant seat gently, and the baby calms almost immediately.*) Do you like that? Yeah, that's good. So anyway, I was concerned that he was going to have to see the doctor after his reaction to the immunization, but he didn't, and it worked out fine.

Comment: The mother's need to rock the baby at great discomfort to herself finally became so much that I interrupted to try to make her more comfortable. Although she did appear less uncomfortable and the baby did remain calm, I was uneasy about having intervened and possibly having undermined her competence by being "the expert."

Excerpt 7

MOTHER: He would only take one breast. He wouldn't take both. To this day his breast feeding is still—he won't take both and, um (*baby sneezes*), bless you. And he never went more than 5 or 10 minutes, which I thought they were supposed to go, you know, 20 minutes or whatever. So I was just worried that he wasn't getting enough.

Comment: It was clear that the mother experienced the baby's putative "one breast only" rule as a rejection. This feeling of rejection by the baby was another theme of the interview.

Excerpt 8

CLINICIAN: When you're away from him, what's it like for you and for him?

MOTHER: I'm never away from him. (*Shakes her head "no."*) I have never been away from him.

CLINICIAN: Even for a few minutes?

MOTHER: Oh, um, what's it like?

CLINICIAN: Maybe you've gone to the store?

MOTHER: (*Shakes head "no" and laughs.*) I can't stand being away from him. Well this is, we're out of control. I know it. He's spoiled, and I've read the books and they say you can't spoil a baby before 3 months. You must respond promptly to their every whimper so that they will, you know, have a good outlook on the world and that's what I've done. And, um, he has to be held or played with or be in his swing-a-matic every waking moment or he cries. And I just don't know how to break this cycle that I've gotten us into. Last night, he was fussing and fussing and fussing all night. Finally, I got him to sleep, and my husband was watching television on the couch, and I put him in his crib because I wanted to take a shower. I went in and took a shower. Then, I got out to get the cream rinse, and he was screaming his head off. My husband had gone out to the garage, and I just felt like, I can't even, you know, take a shower unless its midnight, and he's stone, stone asleep.

CLINICIAN: I see, so you feel like you really have to be there all of the time?

MOTHER: Yes, I guess I do. And also because if he would breast-feed every two and half hours consistently then I could run up to the store and be back in an hour or two. But because I don't know if he's going to want something an hour later, I feel like I can't. I know I'm supposed to give him a relief bottle, but I'm afraid he'll get hooked on that because I used a rubber nipple shield twice—two times—and then he didn't want my breast. I had to battle to get him back on that. He just likes the rubber nipple so much better. Which is just probably a rationalization also because I want him to need me and I want to be with him all of the time and I, um . . .

CLINICIAN: But the nursing, that is what it's like for you—it makes you feel like he needs you, counts on you, and depends on you.

Comment: This excerpt reveals several important issues. The mother's lack of support is evident in the vignette about her husband, and her belief that she must be with the baby all the time illustrated her excessive anxiety and the degree to which it compounded her frustration. It also raised the question about the degree to which her aloneness with the baby was self-imposed because she *had* to be the only one to care for him. This belief could intensify the importance of her relationship with the baby as he became absolutely essential for her, given her lack of other support, and at the same time raised the question of whether her need for control led her to disallow the father as a potential source of support.

In addition, the idea of the baby as rejecting and of her own inadequacy as a mother is evident in her reluctance to introduce a bottle or a nipple shield to the baby for fear he would never take her back. All of the mother's fears had a kernel of truth, of course, and many of the fears are common in first-time mothers, but the number and intensity of this mother's fears and doubts already had begun to seem extraordinary.

Excerpt 9

CLINICIAN: I would like you to describe your impression of Daniel's personality.

MOTHER: I think he's, um, when he's good, he's good and when he's bad he's horrid (*chuckle*). He's sometimes, he's just the sweetest little thing. He's smiling and waving his arms, and I'm playing with him, and he just scrunches up his nose, and he's just a delight, but when he's bad, he's mad, and I feel like he's angry, and I don't know what to, you know. I don't want him to be angry.

CLINICIAN: What do you think he's angry about?

MOTHER: Because he's not getting what he wants (*laughs*). I guess he's frustrated. Um, all right. Given again he's not really crying, but he seems like he's angry and frustrated. And, um, I get frustrated because I don't know, a lot of times I don't know what it is that he wants. I'll try this, I'll try that, and I'll try the other thing, and it's always the last thing that I try that makes him happy, and then I'll feel guilty because I didn't see it sooner that he needed this or that.

Comment: This excerpt reveals that the mother felt criticized by the baby. She experienced his cry as an indictment of her mothering abilities. Furthermore, she expressed confusion and frustration about not understanding what he wanted, and helplessness about how to please him. Instead of feeling satisfied when she solved the riddle of his cry, she felt guilty about not getting it right sooner, revealing the harshness with which she regarded herself. And if she regarded herself this harshly, one wonders how harshly she judged the baby and whether some of her self-deprecation might be a way of trying to contain (i.e., maintain out of awareness) negative feelings about the infant.

Excerpt 10

CLINICIAN: Also, you said frustrated, is that different from angry?

MOTHER: I guess I would say he's frustrated when he's like that—where he's not crying, but that "ah, ah, ah." And at night I'm trying, I put him down to play with him. He doesn't want that. I try to feed him and he doesn't want that. Whatever I do, even I'm swinging him around and all the time I'm swinging him around he's going, "anh, anh." You know he's not crying, but he's not happy. And it's like I can't figure it out, or it's like the times that I do let him cry and he's not and I can't. You know if I put a toy in front of him, and I feel like he can't, it's not where it should be, can't reach it, and he can't get it or whatever.

Comment: Here, we learn more clearly that the mother harbored some anger at the baby for not being clearer about what he wanted, and for not conforming to what the books said he should be doing ("engaging the world" by exploring toys). She was completely unaware of this, of course, but it was palpable nonetheless. It also further underscored her sense of herself as someone who could not please "the other" in an intimate relationship.

Excerpt 11

CLINICIAN: Who does Daniel remind you of?

MOTHER: My father.

CLINICIAN: Is that right?

MOTHER: Yep, he looks like my father.

CLINICIAN: How about his personality? Who does that remind you of?

MOTHER: (*Hesitation, baby sneezes.*) Bless you. Um, his personality? I guess you would say, I guess. I don't really know. I wouldn't say anybody in particular. I know that like I had said before, I know that my mother was angry a lot. She was angry growing up, but also when she's happy, she's happy. I guess you could say that Daniel is like her, and that's probably true.

CLINICIAN: Are there ways in which he seems like you or really different from you?

MOTHER: I don't think he's like me at all.

CLINICIAN: Really? How is he different?

MOTHER: Um, he gets angry, and I don't. I think I'm, um . . . I had told you that I'd been through therapy before and that apparently my problem was that I had a lot of anger, but I was never able to express it. So, I know I do get angry, but I don't get angry in the healthy sort of way or whatever that is. So, I want him to get angry if he needs to. I don't want him to be angry, but I want him to know how to express his feelings. I don't want him growing up suppressing feeling and then having trouble with it later on.

CLINICIAN: What about his father? How is he like or unlike his father?

MOTHER: Well, I guess in that respect, he is like both of us in a way in that . . . I guess I would consider him stubborn, which is, believe it or not, is because I've spoiled him. And I think his father is extremely stubborn, but so am I in a lot of ways. In that way, he is like me. They both sleep a lot. I have said to my husband that they are both alike in that they have two speeds, fast and off. So I guess he's like his father that way. He has physical resemblances. His mouth is like his father's, and his eyelashes.

Comment: Not uncommonly, parents initially respond to the "remind" question by describing physical resemblances. After noting this, I followed up with a probe about personality. Notably, the mother responded unhesitatingly to this question by linking Daniel to her father. On further probing, however, she noted personality resemblances to her mother. What was revealed here was a reexperiencing of her relationship with her parents in her relationship with Daniel. Her previously noted description of her father as "hard to please" and of her mother as "difficult to satisfy" were both descriptors that she might use to describe her relationship with Daniel. These also conveyed her fear of who she was, since she felt rejected or abandoned in all of her significant relationships. Now, things were beginning to come into focus.

I noted her initial disavowal of any resemblance to her own personality—in fact, saying that his open expression of anger is diametrically opposed to her. From a clinical perspective, this suggested that anger was a "split off" and disavowed part of her own sense of self—something she could be allowed to be aware of. That the baby reminded her of this disavowed part of herself clarified a central component of their relationship disturbance. Her own baby represented, at one level, the most unacceptable part of herself, and each time he cried, she was threatened by her awareness of her own aggressive impulses, which she had always tried to suppress and avoid. Interestingly, she also saw a connection between her son's perceived stubbornness and her own. This is possibly a way in which she allowed herself to express aggression, but it clearly underscored the conflict about expression of aggression that was central to her relationship with her son.

At this point in the interview, we can begin to appreciate two extremely important contributors to her representation of her son: a reminder of previous conflicted intimate relationships and a reminder of a disavowed part of her own sense of self. No wonder she was struggling so much and feeling so dissatisfied. The "ghosts" in her baby's nursery (see Fraiberg, Adelson, & Shapiro, 1980) had all but assured that conflict must characterize their relationship and that that conflict involves an unsuccessful struggle to feel close to and satisfied with "the other."

Excerpt 12

CLINICIAN: What do you feel is unique or different or special about Daniel compared to what you know about other babies?

MOTHER: I guess that, I had felt that he has more ranges of personality traits than other babies, only because—and I'm sure the other babies do it, it's just that I never experienced it. But when I see other people's babies, they're always quiet and calm—like he usually is when I take him to sleep. They just kind of are sitting or staring. I haven't seen that in him. I'd like to think that he is smart. I don't know if he is or not, although sometimes I think he's just the smartest baby in the world because I can't believe what he's done and then other times I really worry because he's not doing what I think he is supposed to be doing. Then I worry that . . . I never really think it's his fault. I always think it's because I haven't done the right thing, I haven't given him the right toy or I haven't played with him in the right way or he wouldn't be doing it. Um, so.

CLINICIAN: What about his behavior would you say is the most difficult for you to handle at this point?

MOTHER: The fact that he, he, um. I wanted him to need me. I've wanted to have given him a lot of attention, but when I can't seem to satisfy or I can't or, um. Or I know that I can satisfy him by swinging around or whatever, but I just can't do it anymore. I guess that, I worry that he's not going to progress developmentally because he won't, he won't sit down, won't stay seated, so he doesn't look at his hands, he doesn't, um, you know because he won't, um, be without me, he's not doing the things that I guess he is supposed to do when he's alone. And then I feel like, you know, this is great. If I put him in this at home, he will never stay in a bucket or anything unless he is asleep. If he's awake he has to be played with, or held, or eating or in the swing-a-matic.

CLINICIAN: You're doing real well with him here.

MOTHER: I know, but that's because we're at the doctor's office.

Comment: The mother elaborated more about the baby's failure to comply with her expectations. By not doing "what he is supposed to do," he left her feeling both disappointed and angry with him. Note that she said explicitly that she could not "satisfy" him, echoing her description of her relationship with her mother. She also revealed some insight into the pressure of her own need for him to be a particular way in order to satisfy her. This is a central dilemma in most disturbed parent–infant relationships—the pressure of the parent's needs for the child to be a particular way can make it impossible to appreciate what the baby actually needs.

The comment that the baby was not doing what he was "supposed to do" reminded me that her husband also failed to do what he was "supposed to do" (being excited and engaged in the pregnancy).

By complimenting her on her success in getting the baby soothed during the interview, I offered some measured reassurance to the mother, in part to see how she would respond. In essence, I said to the mother, "I see that despite your frustration and self-deprecation you are capable of soothing and satisfying your baby." Premature reassurance can be patronizing and alienating, as it may dismiss the mother's real sense of desperation, so its judicious use is crucial, especially early in treatment. The mother's humorous response here was somewhat reassuring because she was willing to accept the premise that she had, in fact, quieted the baby.

Excerpt 13

CLINICIAN: What do you imagine is going to happen to this fussy behavior as he gets older?

MOTHER: I imagine that I'm going to have to let him cry it out a few times, so that he won't be spoiled, and we'll get over it, and then hopefully, he'll be a well-adjusted child. But I just don't know how to do it, because I feel, I feel so . . . I'm the kind of person that I just go right by the book. And if the book says don't let him cry until he's 3 months old, then I won't let him cry until Monday at midnight [on his 3-month birthdate]. You know? And then I'll say, and then I kept saying to my husband that I'll get him to go to sleep on his own when he's 3 months old. And now, I just read in this book about when they're 3 months old that you should continue to respond, welcome their cries, and so I don't know what to do. I don't know if I'm going to make him, you know, scarred for life if I let him.

CLINICIAN: Well, you know how the books are. They're all kind of contradictory. It gets you all mixed up.

MOTHER: I know . . . well, that's the thing. Dr. Spock says don't let them cry, and then he says, let them cry to get them to sleep. I just, I feel like, I feel it's . . . I feel like now it's my fault. I've gotten him into this predicament, and if I have to let him cry for seven days, he'll be miserable, and it's not his fault.

CLINICIAN: But you'd like to let him learn how to help himself a little bit.

MOTHER: I know I have to do it. Yes, I have to do it. I know. But I hope that you can tell me how to do it so that he will not be psychologically scarred.

CLINICIAN: You and I should figure out how to do that together.

MOTHER: OK.

Comment: The mother revisited the contradictory advice she had gotten, and again implicitly revealed both the simultaneous idealization and denigration of expertise. She yearned for *the* answer, and she expected/wanted it to come from someone else. Aware that the mother had already sought and received considerable advice, I was eager to avoid this trap. Also, I distanced myself from "what the books say"—instead reframing the issue as something that the mother and I would explore and attempt to discover together. This proposed partnership was my way of redefining the mother's and my respective roles in the treatment. Instead of the more infantile clinician/giver and mother/receiver, it was to be a more balanced adult partnership in which the shared goals were understanding the baby and what worked for the mother. I also assigned a role to the baby of learning how to help himself. This was a further challenge to the mother's view of the baby as a passive enigma—a puzzle to be solved, rather than as an active participant in the drama who had his own agenda but also his own capabilities.

Excerpt 14

CLINICIAN: How would you describe your relationship with Daniel?

MOTHER: (*laughing*) I adore him. He's the answer to my prayers. He's a dream. I just, um . . . I love him to death, and yet I feel like I let him down some—many times, because I'm worrying about the wrong things. I'm worrying about stupid things instead of, um, you know, even I was just so worried that he wasn't getting enough to eat for those two weeks when I was just oblivious to the fact that my milk was drying up. I didn't even notice that, and that's the more important thing I should have been worrying about. And I was worried about, you know, stupid things. And, um, but, I, I love him. (*She is now crying.*) It's going to be a problem because I feel, I don't want to smother him, but I feel like it's going to be hard for me not to because I . . . I, um . . . I guess as I said before I love my husband—I think he loves me, but there's a lot of things lacking there, and I'm afraid I'm looking to Daniel for all the hugging and affection that I don't really get anywhere else. And it's like, now I have a baby, and now I have somebody to love, somebody that will love me, and, um, ah . . . You know I don't even, in some ways I don't even want him to grow up, I want him to, even the thought of stopping breast feeding in a year. . . . It's like I want to breast-feed him for the rest of my life because when he's good in breast feeding it's like I'm really needed, and he really loves me, and I really love him. I don't want him to grow up and grow away from me. I just want a, you know what I mean. I just can't get enough of him as far as loving him goes. Ah, even though I obviously have to go to the bathroom and take a shower after a while.

CLINICIAN: And it's a lot of pressure on your relationship with him.

MOTHER: Well, I feel like maybe I put too much of my expectations into him. I feel already like if he isn't smart enough or athletic enough or whatever, and I guess a lot of middle-class people do that. But I want to, I want to, I just want to be happy, but I feel I just have such a huge responsibility to make him live up to his potential or whatever. And I'm afraid I'm going to screw up and, you know, or that I'm going to try so hard that I'm going to make him neurotic. I'm not sure exactly what to do. I want to do the right thing and I always thought that once I had a baby, everything was going to be wonderful as long as he was born healthy. But there's so, ah, I don't know if that answered your question really on relationships.

Comment: The mother here revealed additional insight about the intensity of her own need for the baby to take care of her needs, and even recognized that he was being asked to make up for her dissatisfying marriage. I introduced the idea of how the mother's needs put pressure on her relationship with her baby—emphasizing the costs of being alienated from a more authentic and open experiencing of who her baby was rather than criticizing (even implicitly) her need for him to be a certain way. Given how much she *needed* the baby to be a particular way, it became difficult if not impossible for her to enjoy one of the central pleasures of early parenthood, the discovery and appreciation of who the baby was. This also was an attempt to reinterpret the mother's achievement-oriented frame of "she is failing/he is failing."

Excerpt 15

CLINICIAN: Is there a specific memory of sad?

MOTHER: I feel very sad a lot. Just because . . . it's a terrible thing to say, but, um (*crying again*), now he's down here on earth, and he has to go through life, you know. I want him to be happy. I want him to have a good outlook on life, but I myself don't really. I kind of look at life as kind of a painful thing. So, it makes me a little bit sad, it makes me a lot sad that, um, he has to go through life and then die. When I brought him home from the hospital, I said to my husband that I just don't want him to be mortal. But I just, ah, but I have to, that's what I have to change in myself. I have to have a happier outlook on life, which, I'm very happy to have him. That's been, you know, the joy of my life, you know. So I want him to have a positive outlook on life. But I know it will be painful, because for a lot of people it is, for everyone, I guess. So that's a little bit sad. I guess every mother must feel that way about her baby. That, you know, you wish you could protect them from everything.

Comment: It is completely expectable for a mother to want to protect her child from suffering. On the other hand, this mother felt "very sad" that her treasured infant "has to go through life." The profundity of the mother's sadness and anxiety are reflected in this lament. I sensed a genuine feeling of hopelessness. Although this might have reflected something of a depression within the mother, it also suggested that her representation of Daniel was colored with sadness and disappointment—that it was, in fact, part of her experience of him.

Excerpt 16

CLINICIAN: What would you say pleases most about your relationship with Daniel?

MOTHER: Just that I have him, I guess. I just can't believe I have him. And when he's happy and he's smiling at me and he's, you know.

When he does something that the book says he's supposed to, it—I just, I love it! When he kicks or smiles or blabs or whatever.

CLINICIAN: It's reassuring.

MOTHER: Yes.

Comment: Naturally, all parents want their babies to excel developmentally, but this mother's idealization of the "book baby" alienated her from her own baby and rendered her less able to enjoy her son—it also paralyzed her ability to learn about herself as a parent, to grow and develop in that role; the constant reminders of her own inadequacies squelched any joy she could have in the process.

Excerpt 17

CLINICIAN: How do you feel your relationship with Daniel is affecting his personality?

MOTHER: Well, one half, half of me says that it's really good and he's to be really secure and loved because he's getting so much attention from his mother, um, and the other half. I guess I feel like it's more the future that I'm worried about. I'm, I'm just so afraid that he is going to be like me. I just don't want him to be like me. I, and I hope that by being around me he doesn't pick up from me any negativism . . . or, I have a lot of fears, which I told you about before . . . kind of. You know I kind of have irrational fears about things, and I don't want him to be like that. I, I, um, I forgot the question. What is my relationship doing to him?

CLINICIAN: Well, how is it affecting his personality?

MOTHER: Well, I feel at this point that maybe because I spoiled him now he's angry all the time where he wouldn't have been if I had maybe been a little bit different in the beginning. Then he would have said, "Well, I know I have to be in the chair, and I'll be happy to sit in here and watch Mommy do the dishes or look out the window." But because of being spoiled, now when he's in the chair, he's just— it seems like the more I try to please him, the angrier he is. Although he's very happy, you know, when I'm playing with him or, you know, like when I was in on Wednesday. He was happy.

CLINICIAN: So, there are good times.

MOTHER: Oh, yeah, there are lots of good times.

Comment: Mother elaborated on her identification with her baby, and her fears that he would be like her. Clearly, this was a difficult issue for her, and she even lost track of the question and transformed it into a more malevolent version: "What am I doing to him?" The identification was something she both wished and feared. She also noted again examples of her achievement orientation with him, which led her to experience him as angry and demanding. Almost paradoxically, this rendered her less effective in mothering him because she focused less on what he needed (as signaled by his fussiness) and more on what she needed (for him to be satisfied and appreciative).

Excerpt 18

MOTHER: And then another time I was taking him out of the swing-a-matic and I bumped his head on the top of the swing-a-matic and then I was convinced that he had brain damage for 24 hours and he didn't even cry then either, but I just felt like he had shaken baby syndrome or something because he had whiplash of the brain. Because, I just . . .

CLINICIAN: Did you really think that?

MOTHER: It's just that I'm not a normal person. The problem is with me. I have irrational fears, and like now I know that was stupid, but at the time I really, I get really frantic over it. And I feel like, you know, I just. You know, if I, when he, when he was a baby, I drove everyone absolutely insane until really just very recently. And even now, I was convinced that he was going to suffocate, and I just— every time someone would put him on their shoulder, and his face was down, I would just go crazy because . . . and I drove my husband crazy because I was convinced that he was going to suffocate. At night, he would be in his, uh, and this is why I was asking you because I, I don't know how to put him down, because I'd put him down, face down, or, and I'd always put his head to the side and then he would shuffle, he'd go back and forth with his face and was stuck with his face in the middle, face down. And I was constantly fussing over him and probably frustrating him because I was constantly trying to get his face so his nose would show because I was sure he was going to suffocate.

Comment: The mother's overwhelming anxiety was again apparent. Beneath all of this anxiety, I continued to speculate, may well be hostility that she had difficulty expressing because, as she had noted before, she was not allowed to become angry. The anxiety associated with keeping her angry feelings out of awareness also could have contributed to her intrusive interactive style. The anxiety might well have contributed to the "trying too hard" quality of her interactions with the baby.

MOTHER'S REPRESENTATION OF THE INFANT

Beyond the important content and narrative quality features described in the above excerpts, the mother's representation of Daniel, as revealed in the WMCI, seemed to have several notable characteristics. First, she seemed bewildered and confused about who he was and what he wanted or needed, as reflected in part by her narrative lapses, incomplete thoughts, and disparate images of Daniel. It was as if the intensity of her own needs obscured any openness to experience his needs. Second, her representational world seemed nearly completely preoccupied by the baby. She was driven by an urgent but dissatisfying and unsuccessful need to feel close to the baby. Third, however, her perceptions of him were somewhat limited in richness of detail, again perhaps because she was unable to experience him as is, instead relating to him as the idealized "sweet little angel" she had imagined in pregnancy, or as the demanding, rejecting, and exhausting partner she encountered after birth. Fourth, the levels of anxiety, sadness, and guilt that pervaded the representation were well beyond what is typical for first-time mothers. Finally, affects were poorly integrated in her narrative descriptions, compounding other types of incoherence.

On the positive side, the mother also revealed some insight into her difficulties, and some ability to reflect on her own experience, or "mentalize," which has been linked to more positive parent–child relationship qualities. She also demonstrated intense feelings and passionate reactions, which was encouraging for the challenging work ahead in treatment—that is, integrating her negative affect with her understanding of herself and her behavior with her son.

PRELIMINARY FORMULATION

Putting together the history, the observed interactions between the mother and Daniel, and her perceptions of him as revealed in the WMCI, the following formulation was developed. Daniel was a 3-

month-old infant with dysregulation, including inadequate and overly frequent feeding without growth problems, who had failed to establish a diurnal sleep/wake cycle. He had limited routines and structure that seemed to be the primary contributor to his regulatory difficulties, though he also had notably rapid, rough state changes that seemed to make his cues harder to read and predict. His mother felt that his irritability was excessive, but what I saw was only slightly above average. He seemed to experience his mother's interactive style as overwhelming, though he retained some adaptability, as evident in his behavior during the still face episode of the face-to-face interaction procedure.

Daniel's mother found him confusing, hard to read, and falling short of developmental expectations. She found both Daniel to be failing to perform as well as the "book baby" and herself to be falling short of the "book mother." She was both anxious and depressed—constantly afraid of doing the wrong thing even as she felt compelled to push him to achieve.

Much of her confusion derived from her own troubled attachment relationship history, in which she had experienced her parents as hard to please and satisfy. As Sroufe and Fleeson (1988) noted, both sides of the relationship had been internalized. That is, with the baby, the mother was both the "mother" who cannot be pleased or satisfied, and the "child" who struggled unsuccessfully to please. Because high academic achievement had been her own area of competence, she carefully scrutinized her child's development, evaluating his performance, and approached mothering as a high-pressure situation in which she was being evaluated (unfavorably). Her misdirected efforts to "stimulate" the baby led to her pressured and overwhelming interactive style.

Because the adaptive qualities of the relationship had been largely overshadowed by problems and both partners experienced significant distress in being together, the relationship was clearly disordered. The next task was how to communicate this to the mother as an introduction to treatment.

CLINICIAN'S SUMMING UP WITH THE MOTHER

CLINICIAN: Let me try to just sort of sum up. It seems to me that the fundamental problem is this: As much as you love Daniel and care about him, and you are not able to enjoy him as much as you ought to be able to, because there are all these other things interfering with your being able to enjoy him—all the things you worry about with him. And it seems to me that one of the tasks for us to figure out is: Can you really trust him to let you know when things are really not going well? Because if you could trust him to let you know then you wouldn't have to worry so much about each tiny little thing that happens. Because if you had confidence that he would let you know in a very clear way, then you wouldn't have to worry so much.

I guess the other thing that I'm struck by is that I don't think you need much advice. It sounds like you get too much advice. You're overdosed on advice, and what we have to do is what we said earlier, which is figure out a way for you to feel comfortable trusting yourself and trusting Daniel about when things are going wrong and when they're not. So, as we work on this together and try to figure out things that make sense, I'm going to be careful about not falling into the trap of just being another person giving you all of this advice and making you run around and feel more confused then ever.

MOTHER: So, see this is a personality problem that I have in that I want—and this is not just with having a baby—this is with everything in life. And I think I had mentioned this before when we went through therapy, that the doctor said that you know I want someone to say: "Look, this is what you do, exactly how you do it, and all you have to do is do it. The formula for having a perfect child is first you do this, this, and this, and I'll write it down for you and every morning you get up and you read it. And I promise you this is a guaranteed formula and then you'll be all set." And that's not how life is, and I know that's not how life is, and yet that's what I guess I'm always looking for.

Comment: In attempting to frame the clinical situation for the mother, I tried to do several things. First, implicitly, I conveyed simultaneously that the mother was justified in seeking help, and also that help was available. Second, by restating the central issue as one of not being able to enjoy her baby rather than one of whether she or the baby is doing the right thing, I attempted to redirect her efforts away from her conflicted, achievement oriented way of understanding her dilemma. This suggests that the metric for remediation should be her experience of being with the baby rather than specific interactive behaviors. Third, I emphasized the partnership between the mother and me rather than endorsing the "clinician as expert" model. The mother's response makes clear that she has some perspective on her wish for *the* answer as unrealistic.

TREATMENT SUMMARY

Based on the evaluation, mother and infant were seen together for nearly 18 months in infant–parent psychotherapy (Lieberman, Silverman, & Pawl, 2000). This involved weekly sessions for the dyad and some individual sessions with the mother. Throughout, I emphasized her experience of Daniel, and encouraged thoughtful exploration of his needs. Initial sessions focused on clarifying and reaffirming the themes identified in the assessment. A second phase focused more explicitly on the intrusion of earlier relationship experiences on her experience of Daniel, in order to identify and eliminate the relationship repetition that had engulfed both mother and baby. That is, the goal was to free the baby from his mother's past to the degree that was possible. In the final phase of treatment, the mother and I addressed other barriers to a healthy and enjoyable relationship. We also revisited the major themes of treatment and explored her fears about the future.

CONCLUSIONS

The WMCI is a parent perception interview derived from attachment theory and research that may be used clinically as part of a comprehensive approach to the assessment of infant–parent relationships. In this chapter, I used a case of a mother and her 3-month-old son to illustrate how to use the interview to describe key features of the mother's representation of her infant and how this representational characterization enhanced understanding of her behavior with the baby and their relationship. Finally, I described how I used the interview to help formulate an understanding of the dyad's dilemma and to identify major themes to be addressed in treatment.

ACKNOWLEDGMENTS

I appreciate the invaluable assistance of Diann Schoeffler in the preparation of this chapter as well as the careful reading and suggestions of Drs. Julie Larrieu, Anna Smyke, and Paula Zeanah about an earlier version of the manuscript.

REFERENCES

Benoit, D., Parker, K., & Zeanah, C. H. (1997). Mothers' representations of their infants assessed prenatally: Stability and association with infants' attachment classifications. *Journal of Child Psychology, Psychiatry and Allied Disciplines, 38,* 307–313.

Benoit, D., Zeanah, C. H., Parker, K. C. H., Nicholson, E., & Coolbear, J. (1997). Working model of the child interview: Infant clinical status related to maternal perceptions. *Infant Mental Health Journal, 18,* 107–121.

Boris, N., Fueyo, M., & Zeanah, C. H. (1997). The clinical assessment of attachment in children under five. *Journal of the American Academy of Child and Adolescent Psychiatry, 36,* 291–293.

Bowlby, J. (1982). *Attachment.* New York: Basic Books. (Original work published 1969)

Fraiberg, S., Adelson, E., & Shapiro, V. (1980). Ghosts in the nursery: A psychoanalytic approach to the problems of impaired infant–mother relationships. *Journal of the American Academy of Child Psychiatry, 14,* 397–421.

Huth-Bocks, A. C., Levendosky, A. A., Bogat, G. A., & von Eye, A. (2004). The impact of maternal characteristics and contextual variables on infant–mother attachment. *Child Development, 75,* 480–496.

Huth-Bocks, A. C., Levendosky, A. A., Theran, S. A., & Bogat, G. A. (2004). The impact of domestic violence on mothers' prenatal representations of their infants. *Infant Mental Health Journal, 25,* 79–98.

Lieberman, A. F., Silverman, R., & Pawl, J. H. (2000). Infant–parent psychotherapy: Core concepts and current approaches. In C. H. Zeanah (Ed.), *Handbook of infant mental health* (2nd ed., pp. 472–484). New York: Guilford Press.

Main, M., Kaplan, N., & Cassidy, J. (1985). Security in infancy, childhood, and adulthood: A move to the level of representation. In I. Bretherton & E. Waters (Eds.), Growing points in attachment theory and research. *Monographs of the Society for Research in Child Development, 50*(1–2, Serial No. 209), 66–104.

Rosenblum, K. L., McDonough, S., Muzik, M., Miller, A., & Sameroff, A. (2002). Maternal representations of the infant: Associations with infant response to the Still Face. *Child Development, 73,* 999–1015.

Rosenblum, K. L., Zeanah, C., McDonough, S., & Muzik, M. (2004). Videotaped coding of working model of the child interviews: A viable and useful alternative to verbatim transcripts? *Infant Behavior and Development, 27,* 544–549.

Schechter, D. S., Coots, T., Zeanah, C. H., Davies, M., Coates, S. W., Trabka, K. A., et al. (2005). Maternal mental representations of the child in an inner-city clinical sample: Violence-related posttraumatic stress and reflective functioning. *Attachment and Human Development, 7,* 313–331.

Sroufe, L. A., & Fleeson, J. (1988). The coherence of family relationships. In R. Hinde & J. Stevenson-Hinde (Eds.), *Relationships within families: Mutual influences* (pp. 7–25). Oxford, UK: Clarendon Press.

Stern-Bruschweiler, N., & Stern, D. N. (1989). A model for conceptualizing the role of the mother's representational world in various mother–infant therapies. *Infant Mental Health Journal, 10,* 142–156.

Tronick, E., Als, H., Adamson, L., Wise, S., & Brazelton, T. B. (1978). The infants' response to entrapment between contradictory messages in face-to-face interactions. *Journal of the American Academy of Child and Adolescent Psychiatry, 17,* 1–13.

Zeanah, C. H., & Benoit, D. (1995). Clinical applications of a parent perception interview. In K. Minde (Ed.), *Infant psychiatry: Child psychiatric clinics of North America* (pp. 539–554), Philadelphia: Saunders.

Zeanah, C. H., Benoit, D., & Barton, M. (1986). *Working model of the child interview.* Unpublished manuscript.

Zeanah, C. H., Benoit, D., Hirshberg, L., Barton, M. L., & Regan, C. (1994). Mothers' representations of their infants are concordant with infant attachment classifications. *Developmental Issues in Psychiatry and Psychology, 1,* 9–18.

Zeanah, C. H., Larrieu, J. A., Heller, S. S., & Valliere, J. (2000). Infant–parent relationship assessment. In C. H. Zeanah (Ed.), *Handbook of infant mental health* (2nd ed., pp. 222–235). New York: Guilford Press.

Zeanah, C. H., Zeanah, P. D., & Stewart, L. K. (1990). Parents' constructions of their infants' personalities before and after birth: A descriptive study. *Child Psychiatry and Human Development, 20,* 191–206.

CHAPTER TWO

Keeping the Inner World of the Child in Mind

*Using the Insightfulness Assessment
with Mothers in a Therapeutic Preschool*

NINA KOREN-KARIE, DAVID OPPENHEIM,
and DOUGLAS F. GOLDSMITH

The capacity of parents of young children in therapy to see things from the child's point of view and empathically understand the motives underlying children's problematic behavior is considered by many as a crucial step for therapeutic progress (e.g., Fonagy, Steele, Steele, Moran, & Higgit, 1991; Lieberman, 1997; Zeanah & Benoit, 1995). In our research we have referred to this capacity as *insightfulness*, and using a clinical sample we showed that improving mothers' insightfulness toward their children's inner world was associated with a *decrease* in children's behavior problems, while lack of change in mothers' representations of their children were associated with an *increase* in children's behavior problems (Oppenheim, Goldsmith, & Koren-Karie, 2004). In addition, we have found in studies of nonclinical samples that insightfulness provides the conditions for sensitive, appropriate and

31

emotionally regulated caregiving and supports the development of secure child–parent attachment (Koren-Karie, Oppenheim, Dolev, Sher, & Etzion-Carasso, 2002; Oppenheim, Koren-Karie, & Sagi, 2001). Lack of insightfulness, on the other hand, is considered as a risk factor that lowers children's sense of security and self-esteem, as well as their sense of competence and efficacy (Oppenheim & Koren-Karie, 2002). In sum, maternal insightfulness is significant for children's emotional development in normative circumstances, and its enhancement is an important goal for parent–child treatment (e.g., Fonagy et al., 1995; Silverman & Lieberman, 1999; Slade, 1999).

In this chapter we describe how insightfulness or lack thereof is expressed in the ways mothers talk about their children's thoughts and feelings, and about their relationships with them. We focus on two mothers who participated in the Oppenheim and colleagues (2004) study involving preschoolers in treatment. Both mothers were classified as noninsightful prior to treatment, and we show how changes in their speech about their children demonstrate their movement toward an insightful stance after a period of treatment. In addition, within the context of the noninsightful pretreatment interviews, we point to specific markers and ways of talking about the child that forecasted both mothers' potential for making positive use of therapy. Identifying such pretreatment markers may help clinicians anticipate the different pathways parents will take during treatment, and may help offer treatment approaches that build on the specific potential for insightfulness of each parent.

Enhancing insightfulness in parents is important because of its implications for parenting and for children's well-being. Insightful parents help their children feel that their inner world is meaningful and that their thoughts and feelings are appreciated, understood, and accepted. Such feelings are at the core of children's images of their parents as a secure base from which they can explore the physical as well as the emotional world. Parents who interact with their children while taking their children's point of view into consideration are perceived by their children as a resource to which they can turn when comfort and help are needed. Children with noninsightful parents, on the other hand, may feel that their motives and wishes are not understood and not accepted; therefore they cannot rely on their parents to contain and regulate their negative emotions, leading to feelings of frustration, loneliness, guilt, and shame.

Shifts toward insightfulness do not only represent internal changes in the parent; rather, they are also expected to be expressed in the parent's communication with the child. Therefore, in this chapter we examine parental behavior in the context of dialogues about emotional experiences between the mothers and their children. We ask whether positive changes in the mothers' representations *about* their children are also expressed in the way they talk *with* them. We close with a discussion of the ways in which the insightfulness assessment can help clinicians in their work. We move now to a review of the notion of insightfulness and its assessment, followed by segments from the mothers' pre- and posttreatment insightfulness interviews.

MATERNAL INSIGHTFULNESS

Insightfulness, that is, parents' capacity to *provide an emotionally complex, accepting picture of the child that includes a wide spectrum of contextually appropriate motives while updating their views of the child* (Oppenheim & Koren-Karie, 2002), is considered the internal process that underlies the parents' capacity to respond sensitively and appropriately to the child's emotional signals (Koren-Karie et al., 2002). The idea that lack of insightfulness, that is, the failure to empathically understand the motives and emotional needs underlying the child's behavior, may be at the root of children's symptomatic behavior is based on a long tradition of clinical thinking (Bowlby, 1982; Fraiberg, Adelson, & Shapiro, 1975; Lieberman, 1997) but has received little research support. To address this gap we developed a research-based method to assess parental insightfulness.

In the Insightfulness Assessment (IA) parents and children are first videotaped in three interactional contexts. Parents subsequently watch short segments from the videotaped interactions and are interviewed regarding their children's and their own thoughts and feelings. The IA is introduced to parents as an opportunity to better understand their children, with a particular emphasis on what they believe their child was thinking or feeling during the segment. Then they are asked whether the behaviors they saw on the video are typical of their child; and finally they are asked about the way they felt when they were watching the video. Specifically we inquire whether their child's behaviors surprised them, concerned them, or made them happy. These questions are presented following each of the three episodes, and at the end of the interview mothers are asked two general questions about their children's main characteristics and about what strikes them most about their child "as a person." They are also invited to share their own thoughts and feelings regarding their children and their parental role. Throughout the interview parents are asked to support their statements with examples from the observations as well as from everyday life.

In order to assess insightfulness the transcripts of the interviews are rated and then classified into one of four groups: positive insightfulness; noninsightful/one-sided; noninsightful/disengaged; and noninsightful/ mixed. Three main features are involved in the capacity for insightfulness: *insight* regarding the motives for the child's behaviors, an emotionally *complex view* of the child, and *openness* to new and sometimes unexpected information regarding the child.

By *insight* we refer to the parent's capacity to invoke motives that underlie the child's behavior. Considering such motives is based on accepting the child as a separate person with plans, needs, and wishes of his or her own. The motives proposed by the parent are framed positively and are appropriate to the behavior they are intended to explain. Both understanding and acceptance are needed when considering such motives. The parent should be able to *understand* the motives underlying the child's behavior, and accompany such understanding with acceptance of these motives. This stance is thought to provide the basis for appropriate parental responses, especially toward challenging or unrewarding child behavior.

Based on this parental state of mind, children of insightful parents may therefore experience their parents as being able to see beyond their overt (and often problematic) behavior, and feel that they are important enough for their parents to try and understand their perspective and underlying motives. Consequently, they may learn that motives and intentions are as significant as the observed behavior, that their thoughts and feelings are important and taken into consideration, and that their voice is heard and acknowledged. Such experiences help children feel protected and secure, knowing that their attachment figure is capable of understanding their inner world.

An *emotionally complex* view of the child involves a believable, convincing portrayal of him or her as whole person, with both positive and negative features. Positive features are described openly, are supported by convincing examples from everyday life, and typically outweigh negative descriptions. Negative descriptions are provided in a nonblaming, frank way so that frustrating, unflattering, and upsetting aspects of the child are discussed within an accepting framework and in the context of attempts to find appropriate explanations for the child's behavior. Complexity helps mothers see children as they "really" are, and provides the basis for a multidimensional representation of the child. From the children's point of view this may be associated with the feeling that *all* their behaviors are seen, not only behaviors in line with the mother's expectations or wishes. Such balanced and complex representations are therefore also at the root of children's ability to feel secure with their parents.

Finally, *openness* is also central to insightfulness, allowing parents to see not only the familiar aspects of their children but also those that are unfamiliar or unexpected, often updating their view of the child as they talk. Openness also involves parents' attitudes toward themselves: They can make use of their observations about themselves and their children to take a new and fresh look at themselves as parents without excessive criticism or, on the other hand, defensiveness.

It is noteworthy that the three features described above—insight, complexity, and openness—focus on *the way* mothers talk, and this is more indicative of the capacity for insightfulness than the specific descriptions they provide. For example, a child's troubling and challenging behavior, such as noncompliance, can be described by the insightful mother as related to a specific situation, and as only a part of the child's personality. In addition, the insightful mother, while acknowledging that the behavior is negative, will be able to reflect upon the motives underlying the behavior. The same behavior may be described by a noninsightful mother with resentment, high levels of anxiety, and shifts of focus to her own preoccupations, or with coldness, derogation, and detachment.

While up to this point we have emphasized the maternal side of the relationship, it is important to keep in mind that maternal insightfulness is embedded in a specific relationship context and therefore might be influenced by children's characteristics such as gender, temperament, or communication skills as well. This point is particularly relevant for the present chapter, in which the children presented with behavior problems that may challenge their mothers' capacities to talk about their thoughts and feelings in an insightful and accepting manner.

The mothers described here participated in a therapeutic program located at the Children's Center in Salt Lake City, Utah. This program includes a therapeutic preschool for children accompanied by work with the parents regarding the children's difficulties (a full description of the program is presented by Goldsmith, Chapter 8, this volume). The children attend the therapeutic preschool in groups guided by two child therapists for 3 hours per day, 5 days a week. The mothers attend weekly or biweekly parent therapy sessions, separately from their children, in which issues related to the child's difficulties are discussed. The two cases presented next include mothers and children who participated in a study of maternal insightfulness and children's behavior problems (Oppenheim et al., 2004). The pretreatment interviews and observations were collected as part of the intake process, and the posttreatment data were obtained close to the end of treatment.

As mentioned above, in the IA mothers view video segments of their children, and in this study these included the following episodes:

1. A separation–reunion co-construction task, in which mothers and children were asked to make up a story using dolls and props about a mother and father going on a trip without the child and later returning.
2. A competitive game in which mother and child are asked to build together a tower from different-shaped blocks. The player who topples the tower is called a "blockhead."
3. A story completion task in which the interviewer presents a child doll who is seated with his family around the table and accidentally spills juice "all over the floor."

ANNA AND TOM

Pretreatment Assessment

Anna is a 38-year-old woman with seven children. Her 5-year-old son, Tom, was referred to the Children's Center due to aggressive, noncompliant, and dysregulated behavior. In her first interview, before starting the treatment, Anna was classified as noninsightful/one-sided. Her responses to the interview's questions were incoherent, unidimensional, and flooded with irrelevant stories and with shifts of focus from the topic at hand to her own thoughts and feelings. It was hard to get a picture of who Tom is and why he behaves the way he does. Most of Anna's remarks regarding Tom were negative, and her description of his personality and characteristics conveyed her anger and hostility as well as her considerable concern and distress. This emotional turmoil pervaded the interview and left no room to consider Tom's inner world, his thoughts, feelings, and the motives underlying his behaviors.

For example, after watching the 2-minute reunion episode from the separation reunion co-construction Anna was asked about Tom's thoughts and feelings during that segment. Her first response was: "He's a hard guy to get to know. He's all emotion and he turns it all to anger." Already in her first remark Anna reveals her difficulties in discussing her son's inner world. Even more significantly, she blames him for her difficulties. If *he* hadn't turned his emotions into anger, she could better understand his behavior.

Hostility and blame are evident throughout the interview. When Anna was asked to refer to Tom's thoughts and feelings during the second segment, the competitive "blockhead" game, she said: "He likes to control and he controls everything, or he seems to feel out of control. And he really didn't want me to be that involved. He seems like he was gonna try to bully me to do just what he wanted . . . he seemed reluctant to let me play." In a follow-up query, Anna was asked what about Tom's behavior on the video led her to these conclusions. She answered: " Well, in that particular segment, though? Not that whole play? . . . Oh, he was fine. I think he was just fine. Really. We were working together pretty well."

In this example we can see how Anna's negative attributions colored her perception of the segment she watched. Anna's initial response refers to Tom's negative behavior ("he likes to control everything") and she elaborates the point and provides the impression that the entire interaction was negative. However, when asked to support this general statement with an example, she contradicts her general negative view by providing a description of Tom as a collaborative partner ("We were working together pretty well"). In other words, Anna's preset concept of Tom as a controlling "bully" was so powerful that it dominated her response, leaving no room to see unexpected positive behaviors not in line with her negative expectations.

Anna provided a narrow and unidimensional picture of her son. After each segment she was asked if she could see in the clip typical characteristics of Tom. Looking at the list of characteristics she provided shows that all the characteristics were negative. These included *aggressive child, immature, needs to control everyone, moody, easily frustrated, violent,* and *intimidating.* Perhaps even more important than the specific content of the adjectives is that Anna did not balance the negative adjectives with positive ones, nor did she try to understand the reasons underlying these negative behaviors. It seems that there was no room for positive attributions in Anna's mind. We can speculate that what Tom could see when he looked in his mother's eyes was not encouraging and did not convey positive expectations. Without such expectations, and without his mother's belief that he has positive personal qualities, Tom is likely to find it difficult to develop representations of the self as worthwhile and capable of achieving positive goals.

An additional feature in Anna's speech was her difficulty in accepting Tom as a separate person with behaviors or needs that are different from her own. She compared Tom's behaviors to her own and found his behavior disappointing: "He ripped up the whole house when he got frustrated. And I can understand that. I feel exactly like him, but I hold it inside, too. He lets it out that way. I never would have done that." In this example, even though Anna recognizes the frustration that is at the heart of Tom's anger, she judges his behavior by comparing it to her own. Since she holds her feelings inside, he should do the same. She understands that Tom is extremely frustrated and that he expresses that frustration through aggression, but at the same time she blames him for being aggressive. In other words, she is able to recognize the motives underlying Tom's behavior but she does not accept them. This way of talking is likely to be perceived by Tom as very frustrating and confusing. On the one hand his mother demonstrates understanding for the motives underlying his disruptive behavior. On the other hand, this understanding is conditional because she expects him to respond in ways similar to hers.

Another dimension characterizing Anna's speech was her difficulties in keeping the focus of discussion on Tom. A large portion of her responses did not focus on Tom but rather digressed to irrelevant stories as well as to her own thoughts and feelings. For example, Anna was asked to think of an example from everyday life that could illustrate Tom's aggression. She described a specific event in which they spent time by a lake, and Tom wanted to stay longer. When she insisted they leave, he threw a tantrum. She said:

> "He just started screaming and yelling and throwing a fit and threatening and throwing things, and then took off all his clothes down to his underwear and dove out the door and went back anyway, regardless. He didn't care. He gets into fights with all of his siblings. I don't think he does with anybody at school anymore. He'll say, 'I hate you' all the time. I'm not sure which of his older siblings tell him that because there's got to be one, and no one's saying which one. But he says it to everybody. Now his little brother's doing it and said it to their dad the other day—I hate you, just because, I don't like you and I don't want you—and he's 2, and I'm like, oh, my gosh."

Here we can see that Anna initially was able to maintain the focus of discussion on Tom: she provided an episodic memory that supported her description of Tom as an aggressive child. However, as her talking progresses she loses the focus and drifts to other issues. First she talks about Tom's aggression at school, and from there she moves on to her concerns regarding Tom's younger brother's aggression. Such shifts of focus from Tom's behavior to her worries move her away from thinking about the reasons underlying Tom's behavior during this particular event, and do not enable her to gain a new perspective about his needs and wishes.

Since insightfulness is conceptualized as an important basis for sensitive parental behaviors (Oppenheim & Koren-Karie, 2002), we speculated that Anna's lack of insightfulness would be evident in her interactions with Tom. Specifically, we believed that her overwhelmingly associative, self-centered, and hostile speech, together with her difficulties in concentrating on specific events when talking *about* Tom would also be found when she talked *with* him. To examine this we observed Anna and Tom having a discussion regarding Tom's emotional experiences.

In this discussion Anna was asked to co-construct with Tom four different autobiographical stories about specific events in which he felt happy, mad, scared, and sad. In constructing such dialogues mothers are expected to guide their child in an open, tolerant, and organized manner, so that the child will be able to use the mother as a secure base from which he can "go out" to explore the world of emotions, and as a safe haven in which he can be soothed and comforted when needed (Koren-Karie, Oppenheim, Haimovich, & Etzion-Carasso, 2003).

Anna seemed to have great difficulties being a secure base for Tom. The difficulties that were apparent in her IA interview were also evident in her difficulties assisting Tom in constructing a meaningful and coherent narrative. Anna and Tom were not able to construct even one full story regarding Tom's emotional experiences. Their interaction was loaded with negative feelings and shifts to irrelevant details as well as to Anna's feelings. Here are some examples from their dialogue.

ANNA: Do you know what mad is? What do you do when you're mad?

TOM: Uh, spank people's bums?

ANNA: You spank people's bums? Who?

TOM: Kevin [little brother] when he gets in trouble.

ANNA: Kevin? When no one's looking?

TOM: I'm gonna eat my food.

ANNA: No, you have to play this game with me or you don't get your toy. Well, sit up here. Come here, Tom. Come sit here. Tom, Tom, Tom, I'm getting angry.

TOM: No.

ANNA: I'm getting angry because you're not listening to me and it

hurts my feelings. You like when I listen to you.

TOM: (*Crawls under the table.*)

ANNA: Come out from under the table. Come on. Come on, this isn't funny.

TOM: (*Giggles and runs out from under the table.*)

ANNA: I'm not laughing. Are you happy right now? Are you happy

being naughty? You're doing just what I told you not to.

TOM: (*Walks up to Mom and tries to grab the lunch bag from her hands.*)

ANNA: No, No! Stop now! Tom, I'm not kidding. This isn't a game. Come on. Come on. Come on.

TOM: You won't give me my bag!

ANNA: You can hold it but you can't eat it right yet. Don't open it. Are you happy about being naughty? Because I don't think it is funny and it's not making me happy at all and you just hurt my feelings.

Anna's negative attributions about Tom and her hostility toward him, as well as her tendency to concentrate on her own feelings, which were dominant features in her responses to the IA questions, are also central characteristics of her interaction with her child. At the beginning of the conversation Tom cooperates with his mother, telling her that he "spanks people's bums" when he feels mad. He is also willing to elaborate a little by telling her that he does it to his little brother when the brother gets in trouble. Anna does not follow Tom's lead and she does not focus on his feelings. Rather, she diverts the focus of conversation from Tom's being mad to blaming him for spanking his little brother when no one is looking. This diversion from Tom's feelings is a turning point in the interaction. From that moment on Tom does not cooperate with his mother; he asks for his food and gets under the table. In the remaining time they struggle with each other, and construction of a meaningful conversation about Tom's emotional experiences is no longer possible.

In addition, Anna's tendency to shift the focus of the conversation from Tom's feelings to her own, a central feature of her IA interview, was also expressed in their dialogue. When Tom refused to cooperate with her questions she diverted attention to her own feelings. She repeatedly mentions that *she* is getting angry because of his lack of responsiveness and that his behavior is hurting her. She does not guide Tom to elaborate on a specific story, and does not help him close the story with appropriate or accepted ways in which he may express his anger. They both remain in the "here and now," quarrelling about Tom's lunch box and incapable of talking about past emotional events.

Based on the difficulties Anna showed in her IA interview we can draw some specific goals for the therapeutic efforts: help Anna concentrate on *Tom's* thoughts and feelings; explore motives underlying his behavior; form a more balanced view of Tom as having both positive and negative characteristics; take into consideration the context in which problem behaviors occur; and above all learn to respond to Tom's challenging behaviors with both understanding and acceptance. These are not simple therapeutic goals nor can they be easily achieved. But some of Anna's strengths as revealed in the insightfulness assessment can help attain them.

The first strength is her high emotional engagement with her child. There are parents who simply do not see the child's inner world as interesting or worthy of consideration. Anna, on the other hand, shows high involvement with Tom and with the task of trying to figure him out, even though it is coupled with hostility and lack of insight or acceptance. The same quotes from Anna's interview that reveal her self-centered and negative attributions also show her capacity to think about and consider her son's inner world. For example, she identified that his need to control may be related to his feelings of lack of self-control ("He likes to control and he controls everything, or he seems to feel out of control"). Anna finds her son's inner emotional world relevant and sees it as her role to understand this world. Thus, the language of psychological motives that are at the root of observed behaviors is not foreign for her. These strengths can be used as a starting point for developing a wider, deeper, and more balanced perspective of her child.

The second strength that emerged from Anna's IA was that at several points during the interview she demonstrated fresh thinking and self-reflection. For example, at the very beginning of the interview, when the interviewer presented the procedure, he said, "We want you basically to help us understand Tom because we think that you are an expert on his behavior." Anna interrupted him by saying, "I may be the cause of a good portion of it, too." In this short sentence Anna shows us that she is able to think about her own role in Tom's problems. Throughout the interview she refers to Tom as the one who holds sole responsibility for all the faults and problems, but here she provides access to another way of understanding his problematic behavior—her possible contributions to it—as well as a first glance at her feelings of guilt.

Another example of Anna's openness is taken from her response to the question regarding her own thoughts and feelings after watching the separation–reunion co-construction clip. She said: "I just feel sad for him. I realize how much I have lost and missed out on in the last year in playing with him. Since I had the baby." Here again, Anna is able to look at the clip and gain a new reflection and insight that could forecast a positive shift. At this point, however, this strength is insufficient and is overshadowed by her difficulties. Such glimpses of openness and insightfulness, even if rare, can serve as a good basis for a shift toward insightfulness.

Posttreatment Assessment

During the posttreatment assessment Anna's responses to the IA questions were very different. At this point her transcript was classified (by a coder who was blind to her first classification) as showing insightfulness, and a new picture of Tom emerged. He was described using a wide range of adjectives, many of them positive. Anna was now able to see in Tom characteristics such as compassion, sensitivity, introspection, and friendliness, and she also described him as a quick learner and very active boy. She was able to support her adjectives with vivid and believable examples from everyday life. These positive descriptions were balanced with descriptions of Tom as a child who can get a little rowdy, physical, and moody.

Perhaps the most significant change during treatment was in Anna's ability to see things from Tom's point of view. In her posttreatment assessment Anna showed the capacity to go beyond Tom's troubled behavior and see what may be driving this behavior. In addition, she expressed satisfaction and warmth when talking about him and much less hostility and anger toward his difficult and problematic behaviors. For example, after watching the spilled-juice vignette, Anna was asked to refer to Tom's thoughts and feeling during that segment. Her answer was focused on Tom's emotional experience during the segment and not just on the story he told. She said: "I think he was having fun, being the center of attention, getting all the attention, and someone to play with, a grown-up."

In some situations Tom's behavior did not necessarily improve, but Anna's understanding and acceptance of his behavior changed dramatically. In the same spilled-juice episode described above, during the pre-treatment assessment, Tom threw the little figures around and made them misbehave. After watching the segment Anna got very angry and blamed Tom for not knowing how to play and for being such an aggressive boy. Now, seven months later Tom showed similar behaviors, but his mother was better able to contain and understand them. She said : "the rowdy and kicking and stuff . . . I think that we've all just been under a lot of stress about having the baby, and I've been in and out of the hospital and we've had to be separated a lot. So he's been really stressed out and acting out." Anna is able now to go beyond the behaviors and explore the motives for these behaviors. By doing so she is able to see Tom as a stressed little boy who had been separated from his mother, and to see his violent behavior as part of his efforts to control these stresses. We believe that such a perspective serves as a basis for a calmer, warmer, and much less hostile way of interacting, as we show below.

Another change in Anna's speech involved her acceptance of Tom. For example, Anna said that Tom's play with her during the separation-reunion episode was very typical. She continued:

"I realize now, with that question, that I guess we still don't play, play with toys. That's because I don't wanna play and have my toy get kicked through the air. I don't agree with that way of playing but he's not about to change it. He's made that pretty clear, that that's the way he wants to play and you know what? Looking at us playing now, I realized how cute he is, how much he's grown up and how much more mature he is, and that it was a pretty typical 5-year-old's play, with all the throwing of toys, which I would imagine from what I know is pretty typical child's play."

Anna was able to put Tom's behavior in context. In her pretreatment IA she blamed him for being aggressive and noncooperative. Now she is able to see that such behaviors are not necessarily examples of problematic behavior, but may be typical physical play of 5-year-olds. It is important to note that at both time points (pre- and posttreatment) Tom's play might have been "typical physical play," but that in her pretreatment interview Anna was too flooded and too overwhelmed with negative emotions toward Tom to see his behavior as normal or typical. It is also possible that Tom demonstrated challenging and hyperactive behaviors at both observations but in her posttreatment interview Anna was better able to show understanding and empathy for his behaviors and therefore is less threatened by his physical play. In fact, this newly found attitude may help Tom, at least over time, gain better control over his aggression.

During the entire interview Anna repeatedly acknowledges the positive change Tom has gone through. She mentions that "before he had two emotions and now he's learned over the last year that there are many, many variations and many shades of black, white, gray, everything. That was a great transformation for him. I'm proud of him." It seems that Anna has gone through a very similar transformation and she is now able to see many shades in Tom. In her closing remark Anna expands this point by saying: "This change makes me really happy. I'm really happy for him. I just know that he's gonna have a much better life and better relationships in life because of that change."

This last sentence captures the essence of the profound change Anna has gone through. When she thinks now about Tom's future, she focuses on his improvement. She expresses happiness with his new skills as well as confidence in his ability to make positive use of them. We may speculate that when this is the way Tom is represented in her mind, he will find her much more sensitive and responsive then she used to be. As with all children, an important contribution to what Tom learns about himself comes from the way he is seen by his mother. It seems that prior to treatment there was no room for positive attributions in Anna's mind regarding Tom, and the image reflected from his mother was not encouraging and did not include expectations for positive behaviors. Toward the end of the treatment Tom may feel that his point of view is taken into consideration and that his mother is open to seeing positive aspects in his behavior. This positive change may help Tom trust his mother as a source of understanding and help when needed, which in turn may help him be open to acquiring new and more adaptive ways of behavior.

Their dialogue about emotions suggests that after treatment Anna's behavior toward Tom, and not only her representation of him, has changed for the better. In their second dialogue Anna and Tom came up with three emotionally matched, appropriate, and relevant stories (out of four requested stories). The stories were concise and brief, but nevertheless they were matched to the emotions requested and were the result of collaboration and involvement by both Anna and Tom. Both of them were focused on the task; there was no hostility, and only minimal diversions to irrelevant details. A short example will illustrate the change in their mode of interaction:

ANNA: Do you know what happy is? Let's make a happy face.

TOM: (*Smiles.*)

ANNA: What makes you smile like that?

TOM: I like making food.

ANNA: Oh, yeah, what kind of food makes you happy?

TOM: Oh, doughnuts.

ANNA: Doughnuts? Why? 'Cause they taste good?

TOM: Yeah. They taste sweet.

In this short example we see a dialogue in which the voice of both partners is heard. They listen to each other and contribute to the development of the story. Anna accepts Tom's story and tries to expand it and Tom cooperates and elaborates a bit. Can they show these features when talking about negative events as well?

ANNA: Do you ever get mad?

TOM: No, I get really mad!

ANNA: What do you do?

TOM: I kick someone's leg.

ANNA: That's not nice.

TOM: When they hurt me I do this.

ANNA: Shouldn't you tell somebody instead? 'Cause if you kick them they're just gonna keep fighting too. Let's do the sad.

In this example we see that Anna is much more cooperative and accepting then she used to be. She does not blame Tom for kicking and she leads the dialogue to a possible positive solution. Tom cooperates with his mother, answers her questions in an open manner, and stays focused on the task.

In sum, Anna's pre- and posttreatment interviews demonstrate a positive shift in her capacity to take her child's inner world into consideration. In her pretreatment interview Anna had great difficulties in concentrating on Tom's thoughts and feelings and in showing empathy for him, but in the process of treatment she expanded her repertoire, and toward the end of the process she was able to portray her child in a complex, open, and insightful manner. This shift was also seen in her actual interaction with Tom. The seeds for the positive shifts were evident in Anna's pretreatment interview, particularly in the few sentences that pointed to her openness, search for reasons for her child's behavior, and high involvement with Tom's world of emotions.

DORIS AND DEBRA

Pretreatment Assessment

Five-year-old Debra and her mother, Doris, were also observed and interviewed before and after treatment. As with Anna, the most salient feature of Doris's responses to her first IA interview was her negative representation of her child. Debra was described as stubborn, uncooperative, and manipulative. Doris elaborated on Debra's negative characteristics and did not show any signs of the openness needed to explore possible motives that might explain the child's negativism. For example, after watching the "blockhead" interaction Doris talked about Debra's unwillingness to lose. She repeatedly described Debra as a stubborn, strong-minded child who gets all she wants: "She just wanted to win. And with Debra, it's like her way or basically no way, you know, that's how she is. And she doesn't really take no easily, she is really stubborn." A few minutes later, when she was asked to support these statements with episodes from everyday life, Doris came up with several detailed stories from which her own contribution to the problematic behavior was obvious. For example, she described an episode in which she tried to force Debra to go to sleep on time but withdrew and permitted the child to decide when and where she would sleep because she couldn't handle the confrontation.

Doris's lack of insight and complexity was not only evident in her description of Debra's difficult behavior, but also in her lack of openness to see her own role in the interaction. Doris attributed Debra's behavior to her need for control as well as to her stubbornness and bad temperament. For Doris, there was only one, clear-cut explanation for Debra's problematic behavior—her personality. Attributing all of Debra's behavior to an inner, fixed entity limited opportunities to explore more flexibly other sources for Debra's behavior, such as her interaction with her mother.

At this point Doris could not make use of the video clips to learn something new about her daughter's thoughts and feelings. Rather, she imposed her preset "knowledge" regarding Debra's characteristics on the vignettes she had seen. When she was asked about her own feelings after watching the three segments she said: "Nothing she did made me happy, because she just wouldn't cooperate. Nothing makes me happy about the way she behaves. I was not surprised by it. And concerns? Again, it's like she doesn't cooperate, and really, she just doesn't listen. I tell you, she doesn't listen."

Doris was unable to take Debra's point of view into consideration and was primarily focused on conveying her perception of the gap between the way Debra should behave and the way she does behave. Her responses to the IA questions were self focused and presented from her own perspective:

> "On Sunday I like to give the kids little activities to do, like I give them math things to do and little sentences around the house, and I give Debra her name to try and like spell her name and her address, like point out letters on her name. But she wants to go play again, she just wants to do whatever she wants to do—or she wants to color them, so until she shows me letters D and E she can't color them. She'll just show them but she doesn't really mean it . . . she's really not listening, she really doesn't care if it's the D or E or not . . . "

Two important points emerge from this vignette. First, Doris has a very firm perception of what a good mother should do with her children on Sundays. She states that *she* likes them to do math exercises and other didactic tasks, and she doesn't ask herself whether the children want these activities. Therefore, Debra's wish to color the letters instead of spelling her name is perceived as a sign of her uncooperative personality and not as a creative or playful wish of a child. Doris can thus maintain her self-image as a dedicated mother and of Debra as the "noncompliant child." Second, in this example we see that Doris is capable of thinking about what is going in her child's head but has difficulties going beyond this understanding toward acceptance and empathy. She *understands* that Debra is telling her the names of the letters because she wants to free herself from the task, but rejects this wish. Doris's ability to see what her child thinks and feels does not become, at this point, part of a broader, insightful stance that can help Doris experience her child's perspective fully and lead to acceptance. It is therefore not surprising to see that Doris finishes that sentence by saying "it could be fun but she is not listening, she is still stuck in the same place."

Doris was classified as showing a noninsightful, one-sided, and hostile stance. This lack of positive insightfulness was also shown in her dialogue with Debra about emotional events.

DORIS: What about sad? You remember what makes you sad? What makes you sad?

DEBRA: You.

DORIS: When, when do I make you sad?

DEBRA: (*Gets up from the table.*)

DORIS: Stay in the chair.

DEBRA: But I want my baby.

DORIS: You can get your baby in a few minutes.

DEBRA: No, I want my baby!

DORIS: Now listen to me, when were you sad? When did I make you sad? Huh? When did I make you sad? Do I make you sad?

DEBRA: (*Plays with the table.*)

DORIS: That's not nice. Do I make you sad? When did I make you sad? Huh?

DEBRA: Yeah.

DORIS: When did I make you sad? When did I make you sad?

DEBRA: When you don't give me a treat.

DORIS: When? Like what? You know why I don't give you a treat?

DEBRA: (*Gets up from the table.*)

DORIS: OK. You can go get your baby.

As in the IA interview, Doris's interaction with her daughter is overwhelming and demanding. She keeps asking Debra the same questions again and again, resulting in a stalled conversation. Consequently, she does not gain a broader or deeper perspective regarding Debra's feelings. In addition, Doris's tendency to be self-focused, which was a salient feature in her IA, is apparent in their dialogue as well. After several fruitless efforts to hear from Debra the reason for her feeling sad, Debra said that she was sad when her mother did not give her a treat. This sentence could have served as a positive turning point in the dialogue if Doris had followed her daughter and remained focused on the child's emotions. Apparently, at this point it is too hard for Doris. Instead of talking about the specific episode Debra mentioned, elaborating on her feelings, and pointing to possible positive resolutions, she responds with a negative and possibly blaming question to her child, asking her if she knows the reason why she did not get the treat. Debra does not answer this question. She gets up from the table and ceases to cooperate with her mother, perhaps as a nonverbal reaction to her mother's self-focus and blame. As a result, we have no details about the specific incident in which Debra did not get her treat, what she did, and how the conflict ended.

When they talked about a time in which Debra felt scared, Doris was not satisfied with Debra's contribution. She took over the interaction, telling her child when she felt scared:

DORIS: Remember when you were scared?

DEBRA: The monster.

DORIS: What monster? Monsters make you scared?

DEBRA: The alien monster.

DORIS: What alien monster? When you were scared? I remember when you were scared! Remember the first time we went roller-skating and you kept falling, like a hundred thousand different times, and you were scared that you would fall again?

DEBRA: Yeah.

In talking *with* her child as well as while talking *about* her, Doris keeps to her own point of view, does not listen to her child, and believes she knows what her child felt. In both examples we see that Doris takes over the interaction, and does not serve as a secure base from which her child can safely venture to learn more about the world of emotions.

As was the case with Anna, who showed openness within the context of a noninsightful interview, Doris's noninsightful assessment also showed one promising dimension that might forecast a positive shift in treatment: her *complexity* in thinking about Debra. At several points Doris was able to acknowledge that it is possible to see positive sides even in Debra's stubbornness and hyperactivity. For example, she said: "If I could change anything about her, I wouldn't change that, 'cause she just kind of lets me know as far as peer pressure moving her when she gets older, that won't happen too much. So I think that's kind of her good qualities. Sometimes." Or: "She has so much energy, it's crazy, but still it is kind of a lot of fun." So, even though Doris's overall tone is one-sided and negative, there are still a few comments that point to her ability to provide a more complex and balanced description of the child.

Posttreatment Assessment

Doris's responses during her posttreatment interview were very different from her responses during her pretreatment interview. As with Anna, her posttreatment transcript was classified as showing positive insightfulness. At this point she was able to portray Debra's personality as multifaceted as well as relating to possible explanations of her child's behavior with both understanding and acceptance. Perhaps the potential for providing complex descriptions of Debra seen at her pretreatment interview helped Doris benefit from treatment. Prior to treatment she was overwhelmed and hostile, but she could still think of her child as having more dimensions then her stubbornness.

After treatment Doris was no longer imposing an "all negative" picture of the child on the video clips. She tried to put Debra at the center of her talk and referred to processes underlying her child's behavior. For example, in response to the "blockhead" segment she said: "I think she was kind of, um, scared of losing. I think that she probably felt that if she loses—if hers falls over and I call her a blockhead it would be teasing her. I think she doesn't like the teasing part." Unlike the previous interview, in which the very same behaviors (i.e., scared of losing) were described with hostility, blame, and no insight ("And with Debra, it's like her way or basically no way"), in this interview Doris shows that she can take her child's perspective into consideration: "She was anxious . . . I saw it from the way she was like up and down in her chair. She was kind of anxious to the point that she couldn't sit still."

It is important to note that the content of the description of Debra's behavior is not different from the previous interview, namely, an energetic, determined-to-win child. We can speculate that had the posttreatment vignette been shown to Doris prior to treatment, it would have yielded a description of the child as controlling and uncooperative. Thus, the difference between the pre- and posttreatment descriptions does not relate to the *content* of the descriptions—but rather to the *explanations* the mother provided for these behaviors. Instead of blaming the child and describing her as the sole cause for all difficulties, she is now able to refer to the context in which the behavior was taking place, and to show empathic understanding of her child's anxious behavior.

Another theme that was repeated in the posttreatment IA involved Debra's unwillingness to read, but this time instead of attributing it to traits such as stubbornness and uncooperativeness she says: "She's gonna continue that way regardless. It's kind of—that's her. No matter what. And in a way I kind of like that about her, because it shows me that she's not gonna be too easy to push over as far as peer pressure and things like that. So I kind of like that part about her." The difference is not only in Doris's ability to talk positively about her child but in her ability to provide a more complex and balanced view of her. Before treatment almost every behavior of the child resulted in a negative maternal attribution, but after treatment Doris expanded her view of the child and now she was able to see other aspects of her. By doing so she was demonstrating an ability to see things from the child's point of view.

In contrast to Anna and Tom's case, the changes in Doris's insightfulness were not reflected in the way she interacted with her child following treatment. Their dialogue was still full of overwhelming, incoherent, and irrelevant issues. Doris did not support her child in an accepting way in narrating her stories, but rather came up with requests for more and more irrelevant details. She also did not help Debra to finish her stories in a positive way, closure that could help the child feel competent and capable. The following example demonstrates these difficulties:

DORIS: What about scared?

DEBRA: The movie.

DORIS: What movie? What movie? . . . you don't watch television . . . what movie makes you scared?

DEBRA: *Scream.*

DORIS: You didn't see *Scream* yet, you didn't see *Scream*.

DEBRA: Yes, I did.

DORIS: I did, but you didn't see *Scream* yet. What other movie makes you scared?

DEBRA: No, I did see *Scream*, with you too.

DORIS: No, you did not. . . . You didn't see *Scream*, no, you would not . . .

DEBRA: Yes, but I did.

DORIS: You don't remember, maybe you saw another movie, not *Scream*.

DEBRA: I saw *Scream* with you.

DORIS: No, you didn't go with me—I went with friends.

DEBRA: I did too.

DORIS: What else scared you? What scared you? What else scared you? What scared you? What scares you?

DEBRA: The movie.

DORIS: You have never seen *Scream* . . . did Barbara tell you about it? She saw it but you have never seen *Scream*.

DEBRA: No, she hasn't.

DORIS: Yes, she had, she told us about it, you remember, she wanted you to play *Scream* with her. That doesn't make you scared if you've never seen the movie.

Doris did not structure the conversation in a way that would facilitate Debra's narration. Instead of concentrating on Debra's feelings, she argued with her daughter, trying to force her to admit that she hadn't seen the movie. The question of whether Debra saw the movie became the center of the dialogue, leaving no room for discussing the essence of the fear emotion. In addition, Doris finished this part of the dialogue with a nonaccepting remark, telling her child that she couldn't feel scared from a movie she had not seen. With this remark Doris put an end to the argument, repeating her own position that Debra had not seen the movie and therefore could not be scared of it. Doris's capacity to talk in an insightful and accepting way *about* her child's emotions, evident in the IA, did not express itself in a child-focused and accepting mode of interaction (at least in this interaction).

There are several possible explanations for this gap. First, it is possible that changes in the interactional level will take place in the future. It is possible that Doris's improved capacity to see things from her daughter's point of view will be expressed in her behavior at a later point in time. Second, the IA assesses maternal representations while the dialogues assess the contribution of both partners to the interaction. Hence, change in the interactional level should involve positive changes in both Doris's and Debra's behavior toward each other and maybe can not rely on changes in the mother's representations alone. Third, Doris gained a significant capacity—the capacity to think in an insightful way about her child's inner world—but this might not be sufficient for similar changes in her behavior. The process of translating this new capacity into actual behaviors may require additional treatment that will focus on the interface between the representational gains and the levels of actual behaviors. For example, Doris might benefit from the use of video replay techniques that focus on her interaction with her child.

In sum, Doris's IA prior to treatment was overwhelmed with hostility and negativism, but even at that point she had a few sentences that suggested an ability to put her child's behavior in context and to acknowledge that the child has a multifaceted personality. Prior to treatment discussion of characteristics that were not negative was brief and rapidly covered by overwhelming negative talk—but it seems that these brief glimpses were the seeds for a fuller capacity for complex representations of the child that emerged during treatment.

Anna's and Doris's representations of their children changed during treatment from being noninsightful/one-sided to being insightful. However, because both mothers and children received treatment, questions regarding whether the children or the mothers drove therapeutic progress remain open. Thus we do not know if positive changes in the mothers were antecedents for changes in the children, or whether gains in the children lead to positive changes in the mothers. In the first scenario, the therapeutic relationship with the parent therapist, including guidance regarding specific parenting issues as well as involvement in a consistent, sensitive, and safe relationship, may have helped mothers handle parenting issues better and improve their insightfulness into the child's world. According to the second scenario, it might be that Tom and Debra acquired in treatment new skills for identifying, regulating, and expressing their emotions, and these may have resulted in a reduction in their behavior problems. Such progress in the children may have reduced the stress in their interactions with their mothers, helping the mothers be more accepting toward the children. In addition, children's better emotional expression and communication skills may have helped their mothers read their signals and understand their motives.

CLINICAL IMPLICATIONS

Helping mothers to think in an insightful, accepting, and open way about the motives underlying their children's behaviors is a crucial part of the therapeutic process. The cases presented in this chapter illustrate the gains made during treatment in the mothers' capacity to think about the inner world of their children. Both mothers evidenced impressive gains in their capacity to look at the world through the eyes of their children and empathize with their children's emotional experiences. We believe that such gains can provide parents with an expanded, flexible, and emotionally attuned repertoire of responses to their children's signals and needs. Such gains can also have important ramifications for children, including fostering their emotion and behavior regulation capacities (Oppenheim et al., 2004).

Identifying specific markers of both insightful and noninsightful speech may help the clinician recognize in the mothers sources of vulnerability as well as strengths. To achieve this goal clinicians might find it helpful to use the IA questions as part of their intake or intervention process.

For example, the clinician may observe the mother and her child interacting and afterwards ask the mother to reflect upon her child's thoughts and feelings in that *specific interaction*. In listening to the mother's responses the clinician should look for markers of insight, acceptance, complexity and openness, as well as the absence of shifts of focus and boundary dissolutions. In other words, does the mother refer to motives underlying her child's behavior, or does she describe the overt behavior with no reference to the inner world of the child? Is she open to thinking in a fresh manner about her child's experiences, or does she use only preconceptions about her child? Does her answer focus on her child's point of view or does she drift to her own concerns and perspectives?

Several additional points are also important for the clinical assessment of insightfulness. First, prior to treatment, many parents are highly distressed by their children's problematic behaviors, and talk about them in an overwhelming, confusing, and hostile way. However, it is possible to identify, even in noninsightful and incoherent speech, markers of the ability to openly look at the child and to think about the child in a complex and insightful way. Such markers, even when rare and weak, are important because they may forecast positive changes in treatment and can help the clinician develop a treatment plan that is based on the strengths of the parent.

Second, in order to evaluate the capacity for insightfulness, it is important to listen not only to the *content* of the parents' descriptions regarding their children and themselves, but also to the *way* in which they describe their children. Both Anna and Doris described their children using very negative adjectives prior to treatment. Their shift toward insightfulness was not reflected as much in changes in the *content* of these descriptions as it was reflected in their *ability to put their children's challenging behavior into context, and talk about such behaviors with acceptance.* For example, in both interviews Doris described Debra as a child who is scared of losing. The content of the description remained the same, but while in her pretreatment interview it was described with hostility, in the posttreatment interview it was described with empathy and understanding.

Third, most of the mothers in the sample from which Anna and Doris were selected (Oppenheim et al., 2004) were classified at their pretreatment IA as showing a noninsightful/one-sided stance—the way of thinking also shown by Anna and Doris. However, the IA includes an additional major type of noninsightful classification referred to as noninsightful/*disengaged,* which is characterized by mothers' lack of interest and involvement with their children's emotional experiences. In the Oppenheim and colleagues (2004) study we found that improvement in insightfulness was greater for the one-sided mothers than for those classified as disengaged. Thus it may be that shifts toward insightfulness are more likely if the starting point is a one-sided, rather than a disengaged, stance, perhaps because of the openness to the world of emotions that characterizes one-sided mothers.

While such mothers speak about their children as well as about their maternal role in a confusing, overwhelmed, and self-focused manner, they are nonetheless *involved* with the child and show an interest in their children's emotional life. This could be clearly sensed in both Anna's and Doris's pretreatment interviews. This involvement and interest may provide a basis for willingness to cooperate with the therapist. Disengaged mothers do not show emotional involvement with their children, nor do they show interest or curiosity regarding their motives or underlying emotions. It is possible that this style makes it harder for them to become involved in the therapeutic process, decreasing the chances that they will gain a wider and deeper understanding of themselves or their children.

In sum, helping mothers to gain a complex, insightful, and open representation of their children can help them think of the child as a separate person with his or her own needs and wishes, which in turn provides an opportunity for showing more tolerance and acceptance toward the children's behaviors. Children of insightful mothers feel that they are seen by their mothers as a whole person, and that their voice is both heard and accepted. These feelings are likely to promote growth, self-esteem, a positive attitude toward close relationships, and subjective well-being. We believe that therapists who "listen for insightfulness" in maternal statements will be better able to assist the mothers in the complex, difficult, but rewarding journey toward seeing things from the child's point of view.

REFERENCES

Bowlby, J. (1982). *Attachment and loss: Vol. 1. Attachment.* New York: Basic Books.

Fonagy, P., Steele, M., Steele, H., Leigh, T., Kennedy, R., Mattoon, G., et al. (1995). Attachment, the reflective self, and borderline states: The predictive specificity of the Adult Attachment Interview and pathological emotional development. In S. Goldberg, R. Muir, & J. Kerr (Eds.), *Attachment theory: Social, developmental, and clinical perspectives* (pp. 233–278). Hillsdale, NJ: Analytic Press.

Fonagy, P., Steele, M., Steele, H., Moran, G. S., & Higgit, A. C. (1991). The capacity for understanding mental states: The reflective self in parent and child and its significance for security of attachment. *Infant Mental Health Journal, 13,* 200–217.

Fraiberg, S., Adelson, E., & Shapiro, V. (1975). Ghosts in the nursery: A psychoanalytic approach to the problems of impaired infant–mother relationships. *Journal of the American Academy of Child Psychiatry, 14,* 387–421.

Koren-Karie, N., Oppenheim, D., Dolev, S., Sher, E., & Etzion-Carasso, A. (2002). Mothers' empathic understanding of their infants' internal experience: Relations with maternal sensitivity and infant attachment. *Developmental Psychology, 38,* 534–542.

Koren-Karie, N., Oppenheim, D., Haimovich, Z., & Etzion-Carasso, A. (2003). Dialogues of seven-year-olds with their mothers about emotional events: Development of a typology. In R. N. Emde, D. P. Wolf, & D. Oppenheim (Eds.), *Revealing the inner worlds of young children: The MacArthur Story*

Stem battery and parent–child narratives (pp. 338–354). Oxford, UK: Oxford University Press.

Lieberman, A. F. (1997). Toddlers' internalization of maternal attributions as a factor in quality of attachment. In L. Atkinson & K. J. Zucker (Eds.), *Attachment and psychopathology* (pp. 277–291). New York: Guilford Press.

Oppenheim, D., Goldsmith, D., & Koren-Karie, N. (2004). Maternal insightfulness and preschoolers' emotion and behavior problems: Reciprocal influences in a day-treatment program. *Infant Mental Health Journal, 25,* 352–361.

Oppenheim, D., & Koren-Karie, N. (2002). Mothers' insightfulness regarding their children's internal worlds: The capacity underlying secure child–mother relationships. *Infant Mental Health Journal, 23,* 593–605.

Oppenheim, D., Koren-Karie, N., & Sagi, A. (2001). Mothers' empathic understanding of their preschoolers' internal experience: Relations with early attachment. *International Journal of Behavioral Development, 25,* 16–26.

Silverman, R., & Lieberman, A. (1999). Negative maternal attributions, projective identification, and the intergenerational transmission of violent relational patterns. *Psychoanalytic Dialogues, 9,* 161–186.

Slade, A. (1999). Representation, symbolization, and affect regulation in the concomitant treatment of a mother and a child: Attachment theory and child psychotherapy. *Psychoanalytic Inquiry, 19,* 797–830.

Zeanah, C. H., & Benoit, D. (1995). Clinical applications of a parent perception interview in infant mental health. *Child and Adolescent Psychiatric Clinics of North America, 4,* 539–554.

CHAPTER THREE

Intervening with Maltreated Children and Their Adoptive Families

Identifying Attachment-Facilitative Behaviors

MIRIAM STEELE, JILL HODGES, JEANNE KANIUK, HOWARD STEELE, DEBRA D'AGOSTINO, INGA BLOM, SAUL HILLMAN, and KAY HENDERSON

In the context of building together, with a set of blocks, 5-year-old Melissa and her adoptive father sit quietly next to one another. Quite fascinated by constructing the bedroom in the make-believe house, Melissa suggests that a set of traffic lights would go well. Her father, seemingly surprised by the unusual addition, asks in a gentle yet definitely questioning tone, "A traffic light, in the house?" Melissa responds with "*I* like traffic lights" (with a definite emphasis on the "I") in a quiet, uncertain way. Melissa, the victim of many changes in her young and rather traumatic life, had been experienced by the adoptive father as rejecting of his gentle and loving attempts to forge a new attachment relationship with her. When we later reviewed the content of the assessment with the father and focused on the observation of his daughter's gesture to reach out to him by tentatively exploring if they shared an appreciation of traffic lights, he could be helped to see that indeed their relationship was not one devoid of positive attachment features and that while Melissa's invitation was somewhat clumsy, we could easily interpret her gesture as a wish to reach out and engage him.

The above observation is of an adoptive father and his recently placed daughter in the context of a qualitative assessment of their newly developing attachment relationship. Melissa's history includes maltreatment and multiple foster care placements prior to arriving in her new adoptive home. Thus, her father has been given a rather tall order, to help Melissa form a new attachment relationship, negotiating the many complexities that each of them brings. This chapter is based on the assumption that by observing the moment-to-moment interchanges between them, we can gain a window into the qualities that make the adoptive parent's task possible—a vital perspective as adoption is widely considered the most radical and most effective intervention we can offer maltreated children. This chapter is an attempt to extend our previous work with children like Melissa, who are adopted relatively late (between the ages of 4 and 8 years) and who for the most part make tremendous strides in developing attachment relationships with their new parents. A question motivating the work described in this chapter is "How do they do it?" Can we delineate, by careful observation of parent and child, some of what can be considered "attachment-facilitating behavior"? Can some of this knowledge (attachment theory and research) then be shared with fellow clinicians, social workers, and child psychiatrists who work with such families, in order to facilitate better relationships between parents and children, the basic goal in adoption placements? This hope may be best realized through distilling the lessons from detailed developmental research to clinicians working in the "front line" with distressed children, whether in the context of adoption or other contexts involving trauma in children. While it may be desirable, it is not required for the clinician to have full access to the materials necessary to actually conduct and reliably code the filmed observations that often lie at the heart of the most valuable developmental assessments. Time and resources often preclude this. Clinicians can gain much, however, by becoming familiar with some of the knowledge base on which the assessments and consequent coding are founded, so that their understanding of the material troubled children present may be enhanced. Some of the time this knowledge confirms the trained intuition of many clinicians. At other times, looking at parent–child research findings arrived at through the lens of a valid theory and methods (e.g., attachment theory) may generate new approaches to understanding and helping parents and children in distress.

There are inspiring examples of research work in the field of parent–child interactions that are currently informing and transforming parent–infant treatment (e.g., Beebe, 2005). For more than 20 years, researchers such as Beatrice Beebe, Tiffany Field, Daniel Stern, Colwyn Trevarthan, and Edward Tronick have assembled a remarkable set of findings concerning the social and emotional capacities and needs of human infants. These "baby watchers" have been hard at work detailing the components of typical and atypical mother–baby relationships. They have broadened our understanding of the minutiae of parent–child interactions in their microanalytic, frame-by-frame observations of filmed videos of parents and their babies. For example, Tronick's work on the timing and quality of mother–infant interactions (Tronick & Weinberg, 1977) highlighted how even the securely attached dyad doesn't get it right 100% of the time. In fact, the rates of misattunement observed in lab-based interactions, when things are "as good as they get" is more like 50% (see Stern, 1985). From this it can be understood that "normal" social behaviors involve children in interactions with caregivers in the confident hope of being understood, and how reparation may be achieved if one feels misunderstood. It would seem that the working through of the mismatches provides an essential ingredient for becoming securely attached, that is, the infant or child is provoked to find a strategy for bringing the caregiver back into a focused interaction and from this learns (consciously and mainly unconsciously) what works and what doesn't. This may be the essential ingredient for a sense of inner confidence, cohesion, and attachment security. For those parent–infant pairs for whom the mismatches are simply too frequent and/or too intense, the frustration and fear (of loss or abandonment) may simply be too great, and they are provoked to give up on the search for attunement. In these instances we can see that defensive maneuvers get built up relatively quickly (i.e., by 9 months of age) that help protect against the pain of overwhelming and misattuned interactions.

Beatrice Beebe and her colleagues have been able to carefully calibrate the sophisticated details of the prelinguistic interactions between mothers and their infants. In a recent monograph (Jaffe, Beebe, Feldstein, Crown, & Jasnow, 2001) they highlight how they were able to predict infant–mother attachment classifications from assessments of "rhythmic coupling" in 88 4-month-old infants. By looking at the features of these conversations in terms of such constructs as "turn taking, joining, yielding and tracking" they were able to define mother–infant attunement in an empirically robust manner. That these observations at 4 months predict joyous responses to the mother following separation (in the Strange Situation) at 12 months is highly suggestive of how early mother–child interaction patterns contribute to the building up of the child's inner world (or internal working model), including representations of self and others. Beebe and colleagues appear to have captured the actual experiences that help to construct in the child's mind an enduring sense of what it feels like to be in, what to bring to, and what to expect from, relationships.

Increasingly, developmental research is able to distinguish between normative mother–infant interaction and mild to major disturbances in this core relationship system. It was this work that inspired the wish to formulate an assessment for the older adopted and previously maltreated child that would yield some of what a microanalytic approach garnered for the observations of infants. These early school-age maltreated children have probably missed out on the normative sequence of intersubjective and interactive affect-regulatory steps that are the bedrock of stable and organized self-development, mental health, and—the immediate effect—a secure attachment (Beebe, Knoblauch, Rustin, & Sorter, 2005; Berlin, 2005; Cassidy et al., 2005). Nonetheless, because of the biologically based imperative to seek out and maintain, wherever possible, stable attachment figures (Bowlby, 1969, 1980), these late-placed adopted children give indication through nonverbal and verbal means (albeit often disguised) of their wish for attachment figures who might notice, and respond appropriately to, the child's wish to engage, slow down, or withdraw and stop for a time until they can reengage. These are "old" lessons from infancy for the well-adjusted schoolchild, but for late-placed adopted children the need for someone who will notice when the "lights have changed" and share their understanding of shifts in mood and the imperative to regulate and guide them, is paramount.

We begin with a brief summary of the principal assumptions of attachment theory and the research findings it has generated, especially as they concern the take-home messages John Bowlby's work has for those working clinically with children and their parents. The second section of the chapter details the use of an attachment-based assessment of parent–child interaction, and its potential to provide windows into implicit patterns of relating, which may then be communicated to the adoptive parents as a means to make explicit, encourage, and consolidate their "attachment-facilitating behaviors." These "feedback" sessions, we argue, may serve to help illuminate new ways for parents to understand their recently adopted child's behavior. Furthermore, the selected clips we show to parents appear to constitute pivotal moments in the newly forming attachment relationship—the goal of the adoptive placement. These relationships are being established against a backdrop of trauma, maltreatment, and, as John Bowlby would have put it, "the making and breaking of affectional bonds."

Our clinical work often brings us into contact with children whose parents were unable to care for them, leaving others to assume this duty. These children have often endured multiple separations and losses. It was children like these that first inspired John Bowlby to devote his career to studying and understanding the impact of maternal deprivation upon children. In the aftermath of World War II, in a report he prepared for the nascent World Health Organization, Bowlby commented on how mental health depends on children receiving continuous care, from which mother (or mother substitute) and child derive an enduring sense of joy (Bowlby, 1951). During the 1950s, at the Child and Family Department of the Tavistock Clinic he helped establish, Bowlby convened a study group aimed at elucidating the importance of the parent–child relationship. Among his many colleagues in this research group one in particular was instrumental in the evolution and utilization of Bowlby's theoretical base—a clinical and developmental psychologist from Canada, Mary Ainsworth. After spending time with Bowlby and his multidisciplinary team, Ainsworth left London to conduct longitudinal studies of infants and their mothers, first in Uganda, then in the United States. Ainsworth identified sensitive and responsive care as the vital ingredient in promoting secure or "healthy" infant–parent relationships and, in turn, a solid sense of self within the child that would launch him or her toward trusting relations with others and a sense of competence in pursuing cognitive and social goals. Bowlby, the child psychiatrist, psychoanalytic theorist, and clinician, drew on Ainsworth's developmental research (e.g., Ainsworth, Blehar, Waters, & Wall, 1978), cognitive psychology, control theory, and evolutionary theory to advance a theory of attachment in three volumes: *Attachment* (1969), *Separation* (1973), and *Loss* (1980).

There are four main assumptions that arguably convey the essence of Bowlby's (1973, 1980) conceptualization of attachment relationships: (1) intimate emotional bonds between individuals have a primary status and biological function; (2) the way a child is treated has a powerful influence on a child's development and later personality functioning; (3) attachment behavior is to be viewed as part of an organizational system that utilizes the notion of an "internal working model" of self and other to guide expectation and the planning of behavior; and (4) attachment behavior is resistant to change, but there is a continuing potential for change, so that at no time in a person's life are they impervious to adversity or to favorable influence. All of these are central considerations in understanding the etiology and experiences of children in care.

The idea of an internal working model of self and attachment figure(s) that organizes thoughts and feelings toward relationships and guides expectations regarding the nature of future interactions arose out of a synthesis between classical psychoanalytic thinking and cognitive psychology. Bowlby pointed directly to the notion that we each carry within ourselves a representation of self and other, and the self in metaphorical conversation with the other. The challenge for adults interacting with children, whether they be birth parents, adoptive parents, teachers, or child care workers, is to recognize that a child's sense of self and others, expectations, and behavior have developed out of the many interactions the child has had, often with a range of caretakers, or single caretakers, who themselves displayed a range of functioning reflecting their own internal working models. The representations in the minds of children who faced nonoptimal caregiving won't necessarily be as smoothly functioning as the internal working models that are formed in the minds of the children lucky enough to have sensitive and attuned caregiving that gives rise to attachment security. Erratic, chaotic, irrational, and often aggressive child behavior follows from the internalization of erratic, chaotic, irrational, and often aggressive parenting.

Significantly, Bowlby was emphatic that while these internal working models, once formed, are resistant to change, at no point in one's lifetime is change not possible. It is for this reason that the radical change when a child in care moves into a permanent adoptive placement represents a most dramatic intervention, and an enormous opportunity. However, Bowlby (1973, p. 201) expressed the challenge faced by these children and the mothers who adopt them:

Once a sequence of behaviour has become organized, it tends to persist and does so even if it has developed on non-functional lines and even in the absence of the external stimuli and/or the internal conditions on which it first depended. The precise form that any particular piece of behaviour takes and the sequence within which it is first organized are thus of the greatest consequence for its future.

A great step forward in the field arose in the mid-1980s with the introduction of an interview technique aimed at assessing internal working models of attachment in adult parents (Main, Kaplan, & Cassidy, 1985). This work illuminated not only the ways in which early experiences of attachment are likely to influence later development and the way parents have a powerful emotional influence on their children; crucially, the Adult Attachment Interview (AAI) revealed the ways in which adults overcome adverse early experiences. The central evidence for resilience, evident in the AAI, is the combination of a supportive relationship with a significant other (e.g., adoptive parent) who communicated the meaning and value of attachment security. Furthermore, this value comes through in the speech of the adult who has learned or earned security, insofar as the AAI they produce is coherent and carries the voice of autonomy from the past, valuing of the present, and hopefulness with respect to the future. This is the autonomous-secure AAI, distinguished from three broad types of insecurity: (1) dismissal; (2) preoccupation; and (3) unresolved grief following from past loss or trauma. The autonomous-secure state of mind, in contrast to the others, has been shown to be associated with optimal secure outcomes in children across diverse linguistic and cultural contexts, including, as we indicate below, in families composed of adoptive parents and their late-placed maltreated children (Steele, Hodges, Kaniuk, Hillman, & Henderson, 2003).

BACKGROUND TO THE CURRENT
INTERVENTION PROJECT

In our study "Attachment Representations and Adoption"[1] we found compelling evidence for the influence of parental states of mind (AAI classifications) and the themes elicited in a story stem assessment of their newly adopted, previously maltreated children (Steele et al., 2003). The

[1]We are grateful to the Tedworth and Glasshouse Trusts of the Sainsbury Family Trusts for their generous support of this study.

study highlights the intergenerational transmission of attachment in nonbiologically related dyads, by showing that all the children exhibited an increase in positive attachment themes from the initial placement to the 1 and 2 years postplacement phases. However, the children placed with parents who demonstrated autonomous-secure responses to the AAI were also able to show declines in the negative themes over time. We understand this finding to illuminate a critical feature of working with traumatized children, namely that it is easier to take on new positive representations than to ameliorate the negative representations that continue to exert an influence (Steele et al., in press).

Our finding of new positive representations coming to exist alongside older negative representations, and the retreat of the latter in cases of children being cared for by autonomous-secure adoptive parents, is consistent with hopeful findings from the adoption literature. Children do remarkably well in adoptive families relative to their earlier experiences (Brodzinsky, Smith, & Brodzinsky, 1998; Hodges et al., 2003a). The opportunity to grow up in an adoptive family provides a nurturing and reparative family experience that can help to redress the impact of earlier adversity (Hodges & Tizard, 1989; Howe, 1998; Performance and Innovation Unit, 2000; Tizard & Hodges, 1978; Triseliotis & Russell, 1984). It has often been said that adoption offers children the most intense form of intervention that exists (e.g., O'Connor & Zeanah, 2003). However, a high proportion of children who are adopted domestically (1) are older; (2) have been abused or neglected; (3) have entered care on Emergency Protection Orders (a term used in the United Kingdom that is an indication of the severity of these concerns); and (4) have had multiple moves while in care. Children who are adopted are thus those with the more difficult histories, both before and during care. In addition, the population of children in care is becoming more challenging as a whole. As more children are placed who show a high prevalence of emotional and behavioral difficulties as sequelae of their earlier maltreatment experiences, there will be an increased need for services, including detailed assessments that can help parents and professionals address children's particular needs. It is against this background that we initiated a study looking at assessments of adopters of hard-to-place children and the children placed with them from an attachment perspective.

The study represented one of the first to look at intergenerational patterns of attachment in nonbiologically linked parents and children. This is particularly important as it highlights a tenet of attachment theory—namely, the essential importance of the quality of interactions between parent and child as the critical feature in the nature of attachment relationships. A main focus of the study was to highlight the specific characteristics that each member of the parent–child dyad brings to this new and developing attachment relationship. The adoptive placement allows for the very special opportunity to observe these new relationships as they develop in the older, maltreated child. A key element in the research was to describe the characteristics of parent and child, partly in hopes of facilitating the difficult task of matching child with adopter/caregiver that takes place with children in care: by using systematic well-validated assessments, perhaps the rates of disruption could be improved. Significantly, the study was longitudinal in nature so that the changes in the children, both in terms of their behavior, and their thoughts and feelings about attachment relationships, could be tracked over time, from the beginning of the adoptive placement to 1 and 2 years into the future.

We were able to learn a great deal about the way in which parental and child representations of attachment interact as the new relationships develop. The families who participated in the study gave generously of their time; they were motivated to help future families undergoing a similar process, but were also hoping to learn something about their child. We were bound by both the design of the study and the ethical approval awarded to the study to refrain from feeding back the outcomes of the assessments made of specific children and their families. Still, we provided the families with reports on the findings of the overall study; they were understanding but disappointed that we were not providing individual feedback. Given Jill Hodges's extensive experience using the Story Stem Assessment Profile (Hodges, Hillman, & Steele, 2000) to feed back to families in her clinical work, we secured funding to extend the original study into a brief intervention.[2]

THE ADOPTION INTERVENTION STUDY

The intervention study was focused on the use of two narrative, and two questionnaire, assessments included in our original study, "Attachment Representations and Adoption": the Story Stem Assessment Profile (Hodges et al., 2000); the assessment of parent–child interaction in the co-construction task (Steele, D'Agostino, & Blom, 2005); the question-

---

[2]Our thanks to the Headley Trust of the Sainsbury Family Trusts for their generous support for the "Adoption Intervention Study."

naire assessments of the Parenting Stress Index (Abidin, 1983); and the Strengths and Difficulties Questionnaire (Goodman, 1997). The intervention study begins with inviting the family to attend a session where the child and parent participate in the co-construction task (Steele et al., 2005). The child was also asked to participate in the Story Stem Assessment Profile (Hodges et al., 2000), and the parents filled in the questionnaires. Approximately 1 month later, once the story stem narratives were transcribed and the co-construction task and questionnaire data were coded, the parents and the child's social worker were invited back for the first feedback session. This session was focused on "feeding back" to the parents and social worker examples of the predominant themes that were expressed in both the co-construction task and story stem assessments, and asking the parents and social workers to join the clinicians in understanding some of the contents of the assessments in terms of the child's ongoing behavior at home, especially in the context of what was of most concern to them. The presence of the social worker was a key feature and certainly added to the potential therapeutic value of the feedback sessions. Our initial inclination in inviting the social worker was to have someone present who knew the child and the child's history well and could serve as a potentially important participant in the sessions, and to whom the families could have continued access once the two feedback sessions ended. We only later recognized the "collateral benefit" of having a group of social workers introduced to a clinical framework wherein the attachment-informed assessments were demonstrated as central to the intervention. Approximately 1 month after the first feedback we invited the parents and social worker back for a second feedback session, where we continued to discuss our understanding of the child's material from the first session. This session was followed by a second administration of the Strengths and Difficulties Questionnaire and the Parenting Stress Index. Thus, 2–3 months elapsed between the time of our initial narrative assessments and the readministration of the questionnaire assessments, providing an opportunity to see if the feedback sessions may have shifted the parents' view of themselves or their children. For the purpose of this chapter, we highlight the use of the co-construction assessment and its coding.

THE CO-CONSTRUCTION ASSESSMENT

The co-construction task is a simple, videotaped assessment of a parent–child interaction. The child and parent sit together at a table and are given a set of wooden building blocks (different shapes, colors, and sizes) and instructed to "build something using as many blocks as possible." They are told that they will have 5 minutes, after which the experimenter returns. The aim of the task is to provide an opportunity to observe the dyad in interaction in "real time," that is, how they actually are with one another. This was initially intended as a complement to the assessments aimed at highlighting qualities of the child's representations (story stem assessments) and the parent's representations concerning attachment (the AAI).

The original coding system, developed to capture the essence of the parent–child behavior in the context of the co-construction task in the original "Attachment Representations and Adoption Outcome" study, looked at the entire 5-minute interaction. The codes were divided into parent, child, and dyad codes and included positive and negative affect, vocal and facial expression, and global qualities of the interaction. While some interesting results were gleaned from examining these, from the initial placement phase to 1 and 2 years later, the results were not as robust as one might have hoped. With this in mind, we ventured to formulate a new coding scheme that would take much smaller chunks of the interaction into account. After much consideration and discussion we decided on examining child and parent behavior occurring in 10-second slices rather than across the entire 5-minute task. This approach allowed us to incorporate lessons from the microanalytic approaches of the "baby watchers" (e.g., Beebe, 2005) insofar as zoning in on 10 seconds of interaction permitted us to take account of subtle changes in behavior at the implicit nonverbal and procedural level (e.g., facial expression, shifts of gaze, and patterns of touch). We also were able to listen carefully to what was said, and here we found interesting material that we could understand as "attachment-facilitating behavior." In particular, when carefully observing the dyads there were features of their interaction, especially apparent when watching the parent's behavior, that seemed to be particularly attuned to building new attachment representations against the backdrop of the challenges that are inherent in these older adoptive placements. For example, we noticed that some of the parents seemed (not consciously!) to be making an extra effort to use their child's name. Clearly for such children, who are entering families where they wouldn't initially be sharing the "family name," along with the importance of identity associated with their own name, this was experienced by the observers as especially salient. For the child, to hear his own name punctuating many of the verbal remarks by the parent seemed to offer a containing and soothing marker, a statement that they belonged together (e.g., the comment "Well done" would be perceived differently than "Well done, Tom").

Another significant feature noted in viewing the interaction was that some parents were adept at incorporating shared experiences, or references to shared knowledge, which seemed to be especially important in facilitating the attachment relationship. For example, when the initial tower of blocks came crashing down, one father began by both nonverbally (in action) and verbally telling his son "not to worry, I will pick up the blocks." The father then suggested with some enthusiasm that maybe they could build a house, and queried whether his son recalled the last bit of building they had done at their own home. This further included reference to how "gramps came 'round and helped us build the conservatory." The anxiety of the blocks crashing down was transformed, as father and son engaged in building and playfully re-creating the construction they had at home. Again, what made this bit of the interaction so compelling was the father's ability to transform the boy's anxious affect to a more contained state, and to begin initiating for the pair the notion that while they were only beginning to build a repertoire of shared experiences they did have some, and that these are what important and lasting relationships are built on.

A third example of attachment-facilitating behaviors we observed was the simple inclusion and use of the pronouns *we* or *us*. Again, while this was out of awareness for the parent, watching dyads who made reference to themselves in the task, for example suggesting "We could build a house, couldn't we?" rather than "What would you like to build?" enhanced the interaction. The inclusion of the self in narrative form in the midst of the ongoing interaction seemed to provide an important emphasis on their relationship with one another, and to be one of the building blocks of their relationship, albeit in a subtle way. A summary of the particular codes applied to each 10-second frame appears in Appendix 3.1. This scheme includes 17 types of parent behavior and 16 types of child behavior, as well as some global codes applied to the 5 minutes as a whole (on the model of our previous work with this task). Before reporting our results across the full set of families we observed, we provide a case illustration.

CASE ILLUSTRATION: THE THOMPSON FAMILY

Mr. Thompson was pleased to have 5-year-old Melissa and her 3-year-old half brother Eric placed with him. The children were placed in emergency foster care 2 years previously because of a series of concerns regarding inadequate parenting, emotional neglect, and suspected physical neglect. The children's mother, described as having mild learning difficulties, had herself endured a disrupted childhood—she was initially raised by her father following her mother's departure, then as a teenager her care was taken over by her older sister following her father's death. Melissa is of mixed parentage (English and African Caribbean) and is the sixth child of her mother. She has eight half siblings and is completely unaware of the last two. None of Melissa's siblings are living with her mother, as some have been adopted and others reside with family and friends. Melissa lived with her mother, her half brother Eric, and his biological father (Caucasian), whom she believed to be her own; the identity of Melissa's biological father is uncertain.

Melissa was brought to the attention of authorities early, specifically because Social Services (British equivalent to child protective services) had significant concerns about her mother's ability to care for her children on an emotional level and to sustain physical care of her children. Assessments of the family home found there were numerous visitors at the house, and there was strong evidence that Melissa was being left alone and dependant upon virtual strangers for her nurturing and care. There was also strong evidence that her half brother Eric was left in his cot for inordinate periods of time, so Social Services obtained orders for both of the children to be removed from the home and freed for adoption. The social worker expressed concerns regarding Melissa's relationship with her half brother. For example, she was showing indications at age 3 of being the "mother" and was expected to assume responsibility for the care of her brother. It was noted that Melissa showed little attachment to her mother and received virtually no nurturing from her mother. She did interact with her stepfather, as he showed some kindness toward her.

Melissa was placed first in the foster care home and was followed shortly thereafter by her half brother, and they remained there for 2 years until their placement with their adoptive family. Although Melissa appeared extremely attached to her half brother, his arrival in the home meant that she would once again have to compete for attention and affection from the caregiver, a situation she had known all too well from living with her biological mother. The social worker commented that Eric was an extremely easygoing baby (4 months at the time of foster care placement) and was doted on and preferred by the foster mother. This behavior only served to exacerbate Melissa's feelings of separation (some of which stem from her difference in ethnicity) and of being left out of the family structure. There is a strong sense that Melissa was tolerated during her foster care placement but the foster caregiver either was not able to tackle some of the problem behaviors Melissa presented with, or chose not to. For example, bath time was extremely difficult because of her pronounced issues with being placed in water and having her hair combed. Apparently, when Melissa and Eric were adopted by Mr. Thompson, it was Eric who was more capable of making the transition and more quickly able to attach to his new parent. Melissa once again found herself in the predicament of vying for attention and affection in an environment in which she believed she did not belong.

Melissa and Her Father during the Co-Construction Task

Melissa and her father sat quietly next to each other at the small table, both equally close to the tray full of blocks. It seemed from the beginning that there was an understanding that the main building would be done by Melissa. As Melissa initiated building, her father seemed immediately to take on the role of auxiliary aide, commenting on the building and gently offering the next block. Melissa called her building a house; her father used some of the blocks to build a wall down the middle portion of the tray creating two distinct building sections. While he only occasionally looked at Melissa, she was somewhat animated about filling the house with beds and pillows, while her father simultaneously continued the building of walls within the structure. Looking apprehensive, he let Melissa continue until the center wall came crashing down, upon which he immediately began to rebuild the wall. Melissa was aware of, yet not anxious about, the fall, continuing her building of house-type items. She was interrupted with a few moments of coughing that went unattended by the father. At this point, Melissa introduced the traffic light into the center of her house and was met, as noted previously, with surprise on the part of the father. She was emphatic with her announcement (with an upturning tone of voice) that *"I like traffic lights"* and continued to build in spite of her father's suggestion that traffic lights are not found in the house. Melissa proceeded to then build a garage for the cars and reintroduced the traffic light into the living section of the house. This time father leaned his head in his hand and did not respond. Throughout the course of the interaction, Melissa mentioned the traffic light two more times, until her father reluctantly acknowledged its presence in the living area and provided no further comment. Nonetheless, this acknowledgment seemed to have a satisfying effect—it was a moment to behold, as one could now witness Melissa's acceptance of the walls built by her father. When the building was completed and the father asked Melissa to recount what she had built, she answered with a list of house amenities, including "a traffic light," spoken with a quiet, quick glance at her father, and the slightest smile, from winning the contest. The intervention with this father would highlight this interaction and alert him to the enormous value of his noticing the meaning of his new daughter's wish for traffic lights (something to help regulate the fast-moving emotional traffic in her new world) *in the house*. We also revisit this theme in our discussion of the results below.

Feedback Intervention

We report here some of the highlights of the first feedback session with Melissa's father and her social worker. The feedback session focused on material from Melissa's story stem narratives and the co-construction task done with her father. Two salient themes emerged from the story stem narratives. The first was Melissa's indication that adult figures in her representational world are not quite present. For example, in one of the stories, the interviewer tells the following beginning of a story: "The rest of the family is home, the child is at school. She makes a picture at school and says, 'This is a really good picture I made, I'm going to take it home.' So she goes home, knocks at the door, her mom and dad open the door. Show me and tell me what happens next." In Melissa's narrative she tells her mom about the picture and then gives it to her mom. The therapist in the feedback session conveys to the father how positive this initial bit is, that she has a representation of parents being interested in her picture. Then Melissa, in her story, has the picture get lost, found, and lost again—"the wind took it away." In this way Melissa avoids having the parents respond to the picture. The therapist/ interviewer (J. H.) explained to Melissa's father how the story stem narratives aren't to be considered actual reports of what happens but rather are indications of the child's expectations and anxieties; in the case of children like Melissa, they tend to show that they are not sure that what they do is really good enough, and that these expectations have been built, in part, during their previous time in care and can take a long time to change.

A second theme that stood out in Melissa's story stem narrative was the tenuous idea of what a family is and who belongs with whom. For example, in one of the stories Melissa began her narrative with a mom and dad, the little-girl protagonist in the story, and a little brother and little sister. By about halfway though the first story she turned this family into two, one living with the mother and the other with the father. She completely rearranged the initial configuration so that they were all quite separate families. Melissa's father quickly and enthusiastically responded in concurrence, saying, "That's right—she doesn't have the sense that she belongs with us, and even is resistant to giving herself up to us." He went on to describe many situations in which he feels utterly rejected; for example, when having her immunizations, she turned more readily to the nurse for comfort than to him. He went on to say, "The feeling I have is like I have this little girl living in my home, I can know her, I can take care of her, and that's it . . . and, I do need to find a way to get in touch with this child before it is too late." The therapists took time to focus on this significant issue, empathizing with the father's pain over his sense of rejection, and spoke about ways in which Melissa could be helped to feel that they were her permanent family. In Melissa's case it was noted that due to extenuating circumstances her previous social worker had not been able to do as much preparatory work with her as would have been ideal. The therapists and social worker suggested that providing Melissa with "life story" work would be helpful to convey where she had been, and where she is currently. There was also much discussion of ways of interacting with Melissa, where one might override the overtly rejecting behavior she expressed, and make approaches that did not overwhelm her, but indicated the parents' wish to be "attached" to her, and for her to feel "attached" to them. For example, the father reported initiating some play with Melissa, who quickly turned away, claiming to be bored. He reported that he quietly responded by saying, "Fine, we don't have to play anymore." While Melissa seems intent on having things proceed on her terms, the father could approach her rejecting stance by saying, "Well, we all get bored sometimes, which is OK, maybe you will feel like playing this game later," thereby keeping the door ajar to play and interaction, and sending a message of willingness to engage when she feels ready.

In terms of the salient features of their interaction in the co-construction task, two main themes were chosen. The first was the father's gentle manner when engaging with Melissa, offering himself as auxiliary aide to her central role as builder. This was linked to his compelling provision of "narrative scaffolding," that is, describing in words what was being built, or asking Melissa at the end to recount what they had built. These points were raised with the father in terms of how such containing behavior would facilitate attachment for Melissa, as his words connect the two of them, laying down the building blocks for how interactions between them can be described in words and form a mutual narrative. The therapist (M. S.) described poignant segments of the interaction that seemed to indicate small gestures on Melissa's part aimed at engaging with her father. At times these were so subtle one could easily pass them by. The therapist then continued describing how the two worked in tandem with one another, each putting down a block, and then Melissa asked, "What about a traffic light?" Her father was reminded of his surprise by repeating in a questioning tone "a traffic light? *in* the house?" The therapist then reported how Melissa asked with an upward intonation, "*I* like traffic lights." The therapist noted that we could see how Melissa's attempts to engage with her father, against the backdrop of many interactions of rejecting his attachment bids, led the two of them to misattune, to pass by one another, without sharing an understanding. The therapist conveyed how children with experiences such as Melissa's often miscue their parents, that is, they don't express the same clear-cut attachment signals that children with experiences of being well nurtured are able to do. By focusing upon the small windows of opportunity for engaging, Melissa's parents could help her see how deeply they cared for her, and try to make her feel like she belonged in their family.

The father returned for a second session to further explore how the initial feedback session had resonated with his experiences with Melissa. While he still conveyed concerns about the fledgling relationship with its many ups and downs, he also reported a surprising shift toward a deepening of the relationship and a lightening of feelings of rejection. Indeed, this father commented on how seeing Melissa through the themes of the story stems and co-construction assessments helped revive in him a more empathic orientation.

RESULTS

The first section of results reports on the intracorrelations observed among the reliability ratings assigned to the parent and child in the 5-

minute co-construction task. Here we asked what patterns of relating we could observe by summing across the 30 10-second frames and correlating our ratings of the child's verbal and nonverbal behavior with our ratings of the parent's verbal and nonverbal behavior. In this way we achieved an estimate of the effect each was having on the other in the 5-minute observation. The second section of results considers the questionnaires completed by the parents before and 3 months after the intervention. Despite the obvious brevity of the "intervention" we did find differences between the parents' ratings of their own levels of stress in their task of parenting from their assessments before our clinical meetings with them and after. We were interested in *any* changes that might have occurred over this short period. The third and final section of results stems from our investigation of whether any of the positive changes in the parents' report of their view of the child may have been linked to particular aspects of their observed behavior in the co-construction task.

Reliability

We achieved impressively high levels of reliability between our teams of raters, comprising doctoral psychology students and MA students at the New School for Social Research. Our coders reached a high degree of consistency with one another. Given these high levels of reliability, a single aggregate (reliable) code was relied upon in the results below. Furthermore, because of the small sample, and the low frequency with which many behaviors (e.g., touching) were noted in any single 10-second frame, we summed across the 30 frames to collect a total score for observed nonverbal and verbal behaviors.

Negative Affect

The sum total for ratings of children's negative facial expression was powerfully linked to three important aspects of parental behavior: (1) parents' negative facial expression; (2) parental touch judged to be nonsupportive, such as pushing the child's hand away; and (3) parental looking behavior. Furthermore, when children were heard to display a negative vocal expression this was strongly correlated with parents touching the child in a way judged to be nonsupportive and parents showing a negative facial expression. These results regarding child and parent negative affect are perhaps indicative of the challenges these adoptive parents face when trying to establish a new relationship with these previously maltreated children. With some children who display negative emotional expression, their parents' affective response is understandably relative to what they see emanating from the child, and so they match it with concomitant negative facial affect or touch that is observed to be unsupportive or by intense looking. Here we might be reminded of Karlen Lyons-Ruth and her colleagues' descriptions of parents of disorganized infants who display either intrusive behavior (like our codes' unsupportive touch) or helpless behavior (like our observation of intense gazing). The parents' commitment to remaining engaged with the child is evident, however, by their gaze behavior and attempts to make physical contact, which, unfortunately, misses the mark.

Overriding Avoidance from the Child

One of our interesting findings concerned the parent's response to avoidance by the child (e.g., through gaze aversion). The sum total of scores for the child avoiding the parent was positively correlated with the parent making verbal reference to shared experiences, that is, making a concerted, deliberate, and intimate attempt to draw the child in. Notably, those parents making reference to shared experience were not observed to have a negative facial expression but did tend to display a host of other behaviors: positive facial expression; use of the child's name; use of the words *we* or *us*; response to questions; reliance on positive reinforcement in interaction with the child; and touching the child in a facilitative and supportive way. Correspondingly, when parents were observed to make use of the words *we* or *us* they were also observed to be highly efficient at responding to questions from the child. When the parents were observed to make use of the child's name, they were also highly likely to be observed to touch the child in a facilitative or supportive way. Here we see the "attachment-facilitating behaviors" hard at work on the parent's part, even when the child was cuing them that he or she was not interested. These children responded with somewhat lower scores for avoidance in the second half of the co-construction, hopefully in response to their parents' attentiveness.

Change in Parental Attitudes to the Self and the Child over 3 Months

Here we consider the extent to which there were changes in the parents' responses to the Strengths and Difficulties Questionnaire (their view of the child) or the Parenting Stress Index (PSI; their view of themselves and their child) over the 2- to 3-month period in which the intervention occurred. With respect to the Strengths and Difficulties Questionnaire (SDQ) and the five dimensions it yields—the strength of prosocial behavior, the difficulties of emotional behavior problems, hyperactive behavior, conduct behavior, and peer problems—there were no changes in parents' views. Notably, 40% of parents saw their children as having difficulties in the "borderline" or "clinical" range on the SDQ, and this did not shift significantly in response to the brief intervention. More encouragingly, the parents' views as indicated by the PSI did change significantly from before they engaged with us in discussions of their child, in three positive directions. Significant changes over the 3 months were noted in the following areas: mothers reported (1) their children to be more acceptable; (2) themselves to be more attached to their children; and (3) themselves to be more competent as parents.

Change in Parental Attitudes Linked to Parent–Child Interaction in the Co-Construction Task

In order to explore whether these shifts in parents' reports of feelings about the child were linked to our observations of the parent–child interactions observed prior to the intervention, we computed change scores. These scores were an index of how much each parent had improved in his or her reported feelings of acceptability (of the child), attachment (to their children), and competence (as parents). These positive indices of change were then correlated with our global and microanalytic codes (summed across the 30 ten-second frames of observed behavior) in order to estimate which parent–child pairs were most likely to benefit from the intervention. We found three areas in which parents increased their reported acceptability of their children, their attachment to them, and their sense of competence as parents.

Finding the Child to Be More Acceptable

Following the feedback sessions, an increase in the parent's report of finding the child acceptable was linked to the following aspects of the initial filmed co-construction: (1) the child showing a positive facial expression; (2) the parent looking at the child; (3) the child making physical contact judged to be facilitative and at the level of a trend; and (4) the child's use of affiliative words such as *we* or *us*. Thus, it would appear that even within this sample, where there was much evidence of negative affect and challenges, those parents likely to find their children more acceptable were already, at the initial observation, predisposed toward positive interactions with their children at both the verbal and nonverbal levels.

Feeling More Attached to the Child

Following the feedback sessions, an increase in reported parental attachment to the child was linked to two initial ratings in the co-construction: (1) the parent showing less avoidance of the child and (2) the child making fewer vocal expressions rated as negative. Interestingly, it is *lower levels* of both avoidance by the parent and negative vocal expression by the child that appear to foreshadow increases in the parents' reported attachments to their children.

Feeling More Competent

An increase in the parent's reported sense of competence was linked to four positive features of the initial interactions and three negative aspects. The positive correlates of an increase in parental competence were (1) parental looking (at the child) in the co-construction; (2) the child initiating physical contact judged to be facilitative; (3) the child responding to suggestions; and (4) the child showing a positive facial expression. This makes sense, as the parent and child were showing signs of engaging well with one another prior to the feedback sessions, which may have made the parents more flexible and open to feedback that could further enhance their competence.

An increase in parental competence was also linked to the following three negative elements of the co-construction: (1) the parent showing a negative facial expression; (2) the child showing a negative facial expression; and (3) the child showing avoidance. These results point to the essence of what can be regarded as attachment relationships in need of support and while we don't have data demonstrating change in the co-construction data itself, the fact that parental competence increased from our initial, pre-intervention assessment to postintervention suggests that perhaps some of these negative elements might also have shifted to a more positive direction.

DISCUSSION

In this discussion, we concentrate on what we see as the clinical relevance of these findings to working with children and their parents in distress. The particular nature of our sample of previously maltreated, recently adopted children will be considered. First, we discuss the relative merits of our micro- and macroanalytic approaches to scoring the co-construction task and the particular merits of our focus on nonverbal as well as verbal behavior, including the significance of negative emotion and overriding children's avoidance. Second, we comment on our results concerning how certain coherent patterns of parent–child interaction were linked to positive shifts in parents' sense of themselves as parents and their reported feelings of attachment to their children.

Our approach to scoring the 5-minute parent–child interaction or co-construction was informed by a wish to look more closely at observed features of behavior, inspired in part by the microanalytic work of infancy researchers (see Beebe, 2005, for a review) and we were rewarded for taking this fine-tuned, experience-near approach. This infant research utilizes an implicit, procedural dimension of communication, including gaze, facial configurations, spatial orientations, touch, posture, and the prosodic and rhythmic dimensions of vocalization (Beebe, 2005). While we were influenced by this approach, it is clear that our work was not as microanalytic as the infancy work, and perhaps it did not need to be. In fact, in consultation with J. Jaffe and B. Beebe (October 2005), we agreed that 10 seconds might be the developmentally appropriate unit of analysis for these older parent–child dyads. It is our hope that our efforts in this chapter may alert colleagues to the relevance of the microanalytic approach to better understand and support parent–child relationships in new adopters and their previously maltreated children.

This experience reveals something about the value of paying close attention to the subtle and implicit aspects of behavior—both nonverbal and verbal. This level of analysis allows for observation of nuances of behavior not necessarily visible to the human eye and forces a level of vigilance to the expressions of affect that may be elusive in more global coding. At the same time, features of the interaction at a verbal content level also proved illuminating as to some of what might help facilitate the attachment relationships in these new families. One of the limitations of our current work reported here is that we have yet to establish normative patterns of response to the co-construction task we have employed with these recently adopted children and their parents. It will be of interest to see whether a microanalytic approach is as useful in more typical parent–child relationships, where language and nonverbal behavior are perhaps more integrated than one would expect in a clinical sample.

The chunks of behavior we have coded and report (the 10-second frames of behavior) revealed meaningful patterns of parent–child relating with two broad patterns being evident. First, we found a rather troubling negative cyclical effect wherein some parents and children exchanged negative facial expressions and touch that was nonfacilitative and showed an absence of reference by the parent to shared experiences with the child. Second, we found a much more hopeful pattern wherein children were avoiding the parent but the parent was not avoiding the child. Rather, the parent was creating an interactive environment that served to draw the child into interaction, for example, by referring to past shared experiences, referring to the child's name, or referring to "we" or "us" without negative facial expressions or negative tones of voice. This is all the more remarkable given the short history these recently adopted children had with their parents, some of whom were initiating recall of the intimacy and pleasures they had already shared. These findings call to mind the insightful comments of Perry, Pollard, Blakely, and Vigilante (1995), who pointed out: "one cannot expect the early experiences of relational trauma to fully disappear as they often surface in times of stress. However, the best chances for getting a child on the road to making up for lost caregiving opportunities rests with those maltreated children lucky enough to be adopted by their 'attachment facilitating adoptive parents.'" Such parents, it would appear, are those who can notice when (and why) the lights have changed (i.e., when they need to override any inclination they feel to ignore or reprimand the child, and instead see the child's behavior as a wish to be included). This, we have seen, may be achieved by calling to mind recent shared intimate experiences and invoking these aloud—perhaps in a "parentese" mode so as to emphasize the positive, relationship-building quality to these family experiences. Other parental behaviors apparently important in facilitating change include responding to questions from the child and refusing to get stuck in negative facial emotional exchanges.

In terms of the title this chapter, elicited by the evocative request of Melissa, who requested traffic lights as interesting additions to the house she and adoptive father were building, adoptive parents should be encouraged to recognize the context out of which their children's sometimes peculiar and obstinate requests come from—deeply felt needs for understanding and support. Melissa's request calls to mind experiences of driving a car when we are sometimes stopped at a dysfunctional light "stuck" on red. After a reasonable period of time, we wisely conclude that we should advance slowly and carefully, as there are risks involved in going through the red light, but if we failed to recognize the special "dysfunctional" context of the message, we would stay put and not advance anywhere. These children want to advance but need the help of their adoptive parents, who, in turn, may need the insight of the therapist to orient them toward understanding the emotional signals emanating from their late-adopted children and the need to ignore the red light, override the avoidance, respond to questions, and reinforce the new family script in the process of being written.

This set of clinical tools informed the brief feedback provided to the parents participating in the intervention and, with some parents, had a positive effect. For example, engaging with some parents about the possible meaning their child's behavior or bringing into clearer view specific features of their interaction with their child may have prompted them to see their child (and themselves) in new ways, at once more realistic and more hopeful. This view is bolstered by the findings of correlates with parents' increasing sense of competence and reported acceptability of their children. Taken together, these findings highlight how much more positive a parent's reported feelings of the parent–child relationship are likely to be if the child is able to show, in even very subtle ways (as with a gentle touching of the parent), that the parent is needed. Expressions of dependence by children on their adoptive parents may be fundamental to eliciting a fondness for the child, and a corresponding belief by the parents in their own competence. In clinical work with adoptive parents who find it hard to believe that their recently placed children need or want them, it may be vital to point out the disguised ways in which their children are conveying this very need and want. As noted in the early sections of this chapter, there is growing evidence for the usefulness of "overriding" what appear to be the attachment-deflecting behaviors that such children express (Dozier, Higley, Albus, & Nutter, 2002; Lieberman, 2003; Marvin, Cooper, Hoffman, & Powell, 2002). Despite a child's display of avoidant behaviors toward the parent, parents who can find their way toward engaging with their children and letting them know that they are "in mind" help to consolidate these relationships. This does stand in some contrast to the attachment research that instead highlights the need to follow the child's lead and not intrude into the child's space. For example, one of the paths leading to disorganized attachment in infants is maternal intrusiveness (Lyons-Ruth & Jacobvitz, 1999). However, overriding the child's seeming disinterest in attachment overtures by the parent—when done with sensitivity—is not parental intrusiveness. Still, this does suggest that there exists a delicate balance in helping adoptive parents make their attachment presence felt, but not go so far as to intrude.

In the work reported here, a vital element of the parents' strategies for overriding children's avoidance involved verbal responses, such using the child's name, the use of pronouns such as *we* or *us*, and reference to shared past experience or reference points. The verbal nature of this strategy invites consideration of whether parents' own reflections on their personal history would be correlates of this relationship-building strategy. That is, while we did not have access to AAIs for the parents who participated in the work reported here, we would expect references to shared experiences in the co-construction task to come to the parents' minds most easily if their AAIs were classified autonomous-secure and coherent. We don't imagine that the didactic use of the child's name and the use of *we/us* in and of themselves promotes attachment, but rather, we would anticipate this outcome when these references to shared experience are made by a parent whose state of mind is especially attuned to, and valuing of, attachment. However, we would still explore the usefulness of transmitting this message to adoptive and foster parents in the context of work with them aimed at promoting secure attachment relationships with children in their care.

Moving forward with our inspiration from the infancy researchers, a potential next step would be to share with the parent examples of the filmed interactions with their children. Care would need to be taken, as is the norm in parent–infant work, to carefully select the vignettes to be used as catalysts for promoting parents' understanding of themselves and their children. We are aware of one colleague who has ventured toward incorporating this microanalytic approach with older (than infants) clinic-referred children, where an element of film-based feedback forms the basis of the intervention (Downing, 2004). In our future work, we therefore plan to incorporate the brief 5-minute filmed observation discussed here, and further explore how the ways parents and children negotiate this task may deliver powerful clues as to the nature of their relationship to one another, and the likelihood of their being able to benefit from feedback in a therapeutic context.

To summarize the potential take-home messages of the work in this chapter, there are three that present themselves: (1) attachment-facilitating behaviors were evident in the adoptive parents who were able to maintain a positive emotional exchange (at the nonverbal level of facial expression), and the verbal level involving use of the child's name, reference to *we* or *us*, and reference to shared past experiences *even when the duration of their shared history is no more than a few months;* (2) subtle expressions of avoidance by the parent are a potential indicator of poor attachment outcome; and (3) avoidance from maltreated children is to be expected and if it can be "overridden" (i.e., if the parent is helped not to feel rejected) the relationship is likely to flourish.

ACKNOWLEDGMENTS

We would like to acknowledge the generosity of the Tedworth Charitable, Glasshouse, and Headley Trusts from the Sainsbury Family Trusts. As well, we are indebted to the research team who coded the co-construction interactions.

REFERENCES

Abidin, R. (1983). *Parenting Stress Index Test Manual.* Charlottesville, VA: Pediatric Psychology Press.

Ainsworth, M., Blehar, M., Waters, E., & Wall, S. (1978). *Patterns of attachment: A psychological study of the Strange Situation.* Hillsdale, NJ: Erlbaum.

Beebe, B. (2005). Mother–infant research informs mother–infant treatment. *Psychoanalytic Study of the Child, 60,* 7–46.

Beebe, B., Knoblauch, S., Rustin, J., & Sorter, D. (2005). *Forms of intersubjectivity in infant research and adult treatment.* New York: Other Press.

Berlin, L. J. (2005). Interventions to enhance early attachments: The state of the field today. In L. J. Berlin, Y. Ziv, L. Amaya-Jackson, & M. T. Greenberg (Eds.), *Enhancing early attachments: Theory, research, intervention, and policy* (pp. 3–33). New York: Guilford Press.

Bowlby, J. (1951). *Maternal care and mental health: A report prepared on behalf of the World Health Organization as a contribution to the United Nations programme for the welfare of homeless children.* Geneva: World Health Organization.

Bowlby, J. (1969). *Attachment and loss: Vol. 1. Attachment.* New York: Basic Books.

Bowlby, J. (1973). *Attachment and loss. Vol. 2. Separation: Anxiety and anger.* New York: Basic Books.

Bowlby, J. (1980). *Attachment and loss. Vol. 3. Loss.* New York: Basic Books.

Bowlby, J. (1988). *A secure base: Clinical applications of attachment theory.* New York: Basic Books

Brodzinsky, D. M., Smith, D. W., & Brodzinsky, A. (1998). *Children's adjustment to adoption: developmental and clinical issues.* Thousand Oaks, CA: Sage.

Cassidy, J., Woodhouse, S. S., Cooper, G., Hoffman, K., Powell, B., & Rodenberg, M. (2005). Examination of the precursors of infant attachment security: Implications for early intervention and intervention research. In L. J. Berlin, Y. Ziv, L. Amaya-Jackson, & M. T. Greenberg (Eds.), *Enhancing early attachments: Theory, research, intervention, and policy.* (pp. 34–60). New York: Guilford Press

Downing, G. (2004). Emotion, body, and parent–infant interaction. In J. Nadel & D. Muir (Eds.), *Emotional development: Recent research advances* (pp. 429–449). Oxford, UK: Oxford University Press.

Dozier, M., Higley, E., Albus, K. E., & Nutter, A. (2002). Intervening with foster infants' caregivers: Targeting three critical needs. *Infant Mental Health Journal, 23*(5), 541–554.

Goodman, R. (1997). The Strengths and Difficulties Questionnaire: A research note. *Journal of Child Psychology and Psychiatry, 38,* 581–586.

Hodges, J., Steele, M., Hillman, S., & Henderson, K. (2002). *Coding Manual for Story Stem Assessment Profile.* Unpublished manuscript, the Anna Freud Centre, London.

Hodges, J., Steele, M., Hillman, S., & Henderson, K. (2003a). Mental representations and defences in severely maltreated children: A story stem battery and rating system for clinical assessment and research applications. In R. Emde, D. Wolf, & D. Oppenheim (Eds.), *Revealing the inner worlds of young children: The MacArthur Story Stem Battery and parent–child narratives* (pp. 240–267). Oxford, UK: Oxford University Press.

Hodges, J., Steele, M., Hillman, S., Henderson, K., & Kaniuk, J. (2003b). Changes in attachment representations over the first year of adoptive placement: Narratives of maltreated children. *Journal of Child Clinical Psychology, 8,* 351–368.

Hodges, J., & Tizard, B. (1989). Social and family relationships of ex-institutional adolescents. *Journal of Child Psychology and Psychiatry, 30,* 77–97.

Howe, D. (1998). *Patterns of adoption: Nature, nurture, and psychosocial development.* Oxford, UK: Blackwell Science.

Jaffe, J., Beebe, B., Feldstein, S., Crown, C. L., & Jasnow, M. D. (2001). Rhythms of dialogue in infancy: Coordinated timing in development. *Monographs of the Society for Research in Child Development, 66*(2), 1–132.

Lieberman, A. (2003). The treatment of attachment disorder in infancy and early childhood: Reflections from clinical intervention with later adopted foster care children. *Attachment and Human Development, 5,* 279–282.

Lyons-Ruth, K., & Jacobvitz, D. (1999). Attachment disorganization: Unresolved loss, relational violence, and lapses in behavioral and attentional strategies. In J. Cassidy & P. R. Shaver (Eds.), *Handbook of attachment: Theory, research, and clinical applications* (pp. 520–554). New York: Guilford Press.

Main, M., Kaplan, N., & Cassidy, J. (1985). Security in infancy, childhood, and adulthood: A move to the level of representation. In I. Bretherton & E. Waters (Eds.), Growing points of attachment theory and research. *Monographs of the Society for Research in Child Development, 50*(1–2, Serial No. 209), 66–104.

Marvin, R., Cooper, G., Hoffman, K., & Powell, B. (2002). The Circle of Security Project: Attachment-based intervention with caregiver–preschool child dyads. *Attachment and Human Development, 4*(1), 107–124.

O'Connor, T. G., & Zeanah, C. H. (2003). Attachment disorders: Assessment strategies and treatment approaches. *Attachment and Human Development, 5,* 223–244.

Performance and Innovation Unit. (2000). *Prime Minister's Review of Adoption.* London: Cabinet Office. Available online at http://www.doh.gov.uk/adoption/

Perry B. D., Pollard, R., Blakely, W., & Vigilante, D. (1995). Childhood trauma, the neurobiology of adaptation and "use dependent" development of the brain: How "states" become "traits." *Infant Mental Health Journal, 16*(4), 271–291.

Steele, M., D'Agostino, D., & Blom, I. (2005). *The co-construction coding manual: Verbal and non-verbal behavior.* Unpublished manuscript.

Steele, M., Henderson, K., Hodges, J., Kaniuk, J., Hillman, S., & Steele, H. (in press). In the best interests of the late-placed child: A report from the attachment representations and adoption outcome study. In L. C. Mayes, P. Fonagy, & M. Target (Eds.), *Developmental science and psychoanalysis : Integration and innovation.* London: Karnac Books.

Steele, M., Hodges, J., Kaniuk, J., Hillman, S., & Henderson, K. (2003). Attachment representations and adoption: Associations between maternal states of mind and emotion narratives in previously maltreated children. *Journal of Child Psychotherapy, 29,* 187–205.

Stern, D. (1985). *The interpersonal world of the infant.* New York: International University Press.

Tizard, B., & Hodges, J. (1978). The effect of early institutional rearing on the development of eight-year-old children. *Journal of Child Psychology and Psychiatry, 19,* 99–118.

Triseliotis, J., & Russell, J. (1984). *Hard to place: The outcome of adoption and residential care.* London: Heinemann.

Tronick, E., & Weinberg, M. (1997). Depressed mothers and infants: Failure to form dyadic states of consciousness. In L. Murray & P. J. Cooper (Eds.), *Postpartum depression and child development* (pp. 54–81). New York: Guilford Press.

Appendix 3.1. Summary of Co-Construction Coding Scheme Manual

Parent Nonverbal Ratings

These codes measure the effectiveness of the parent's nonverbal communication skills, including such things as facial expression, tone of voice, gestures, spatial arrangements, patterns of touch, and other nonverbal features.

- *Parent seeks physical proximity*—how close and available the parent is in relation to the child.
- *Parent avoids physical proximity*—how unavailable or distant the parent is from the child.
- *Looking behavior—quantitatively* measures parent eye contact with the child.
- *Facial expression (positive)*—indicates parent's enthusiasm.
- *Facial expression (negative)*—indicates parent's lack of enthusiasm.
- *Gestures*—whether or not the parent uses gestures to aid in the interaction with the child.
- *Patterns of touch (supportive)*—is parent able to gauge the child's needs and respond to cues with the appropriate touch?
- *Patterns of touch (nonsupportive)*—is parent incapable of gauging child's needs and responding with inappropriate touch?

Parent Verbal Ratings

These codes measure the parent's use of verbal skills when communicating with the child during the entire interaction with emphasis on how the parent uses his or her voice and words to convey a message through pronunciation and emotion.

- *Vocal expression (positive)*—positive vocal expression—its range, intensity, frequency, and upward intonation.
- *Vocal expression (neutral)*—neutral vocal expression—its range, intensity, frequency, and lack of intonation.
- *Vocal expression (negative)*—negative vocal expression—its range, intensity, frequency, and downward intonation.
- *Use of child's name—quantitatively* measures whether the parent uses the child's name during the interaction.
- *Use of pronoun "we" or "us"—quantitatively* measures whether the parent uses the word *we* or *us*.
- *Response to questions*—whether parent responds to the child's questions during the interaction.
- *Asks questions/makes suggestions*—whether parent asks questions or makes suggestions and takes initiatives.

- *Positive verbal reinforcement*—whether the parent uses positive reinforcement during the interaction.
- *Reference to shared experiences*—whether the parent references a previous shared experience during the interaction.

Parent Global Ratings

These codes measure the parent's overall demeanor and response to the child during the building interaction. These codes include how the demeanor is both reflected and expressed.

- *Positive quality of demeanor*—measures the *positive* affect the parent has and shows toward the child. This includes warmth, smiling, laughing, praise, enjoyment, reference to the child, and any behavior the coder feels is positive for the child.
- *Neutral quality of demeanor*—measures the *neutral* affect the parent has and shows toward the child. This includes distance, withdrawal, flatness, disinterest, lack of reference to the child, and any behavior the coder feels indicates distance from the child.
- *Negative quality of demeanor*—measures the *negative* affect the parent has and shows toward the child. This includes criticism, contempt, tension, anger, annoyance, and any behavior that the coder feels is negative for the child.
- *Encouraging behavior*—measures how encouraging the parent is during the interaction with the child. An *encouraging* parent will show higher levels of initiative and suggestions and generally be more involved in the task and the child's input.
- *Controlling behavior*—measures how controlling the parent is during the interaction with the child. A *controlling* parent will show higher levels of involvement *without* regard to the child's input, to the point of excluding the child.
- *Sensitivity to child*—measures how sensitive the parent is to needs of the child and the ease with which they are able to adjust their own behavior to meet those needs.
- *Response to blocks falling*—measures the parent response to an accidental/ purposeful collapse of the blocks. *For this code only*, code response as: 0 = none, 1 = positive, 2 = neutral, 3 = negative.

Child Nonverbal Ratings

These codes measure the child's nonverbal communication skills, which include facial expression, tone of voice, gestures, spatial arrangements, patterns of touch, and other nonverbal acts.

- *Child seeks physical proximity*—how close the child is to the parent.
- *Child avoids physical proximity*—how far and distant the child is from the parent.

- *Looking behavior—quantitatively* measures how often the child makes eye contact and looks directly at the parent.
- *Facial expression* (positive)—positive expressions used by the child that indicate child's enthusiasm.
- *Facial expression* (negative)—negative expressions used by the child indicating child's lack of enthusiasm.
- *Gestures*—whether the child uses gestures to obtain support and/or guidance in the interaction.
- *Patterns of touch* (facilitative)—whether the child uses touch to facilitate the interaction with the parent.
- *Patterns of touch* (disruptive)—whether the child uses touch to disrupt the interaction with the parent.

Child Verbal Ratings

These codes measure the child's use of verbal skills when communicating with the parent during the entire interaction. Emphasis is on the use of voice and words to convey a message through pronunciation and emotion.

- *Vocal expression (positive)*—positive vocal expression—its range, intensity, frequency, and upward intonation.
- *Vocal expression (neutral)*—neutral vocal expression—its range, intensity, frequency, and lack of any intonation.
- *Vocal expression (negative)*—negative vocal expression—its range, intensity, frequency, and downward intonation.
- *Use of parent's name (title, first name, etc.)*—Mother, Mommy, Mom, Father, Daddy, Dad.
- *Use of pronoun "we" or "us"*—*quantitatively* measures use of the word *we* or *us*.
- *Response to questions*—whether the child responds to the parent's questions during the interaction.
- *Response to suggestions/initiatives*—whether the child responds to the parent's suggestions and initiatives.
- *Take initiatives and make suggestions*—whether the child makes suggestions and takes initiatives.

Child Global Ratings

These codes measure the child's overall demeanor and response to the parent during the building interaction and how the demeanor is both reflected and expressed.

- *Positive quality of demeanor*—includes warmth, smiling, laughing, enjoyment—any behavior coder feels is positive.
- *Neutral quality of demeanor*—includes distance, withdrawal, flatness, disinterest—any behavior that shows distance.

- *Negative quality of demeanor*—includes anxiety, tension, anger, distance, annoyance, irritability, criticism.
- *Controlling behavior*—will show higher levels of involvement *without* regard to the parent's input, to the point of excluding the parent.
- *Attention/focus*—child's sustained continuation of attention during the task.
- *Response to bricks falling*—child's response to accidental/purposeful collapse of the blocks onto the table or the floor. *For this code only*, code response as: 0 = none, 1 = positive, 2 = neutral, 3 = negative.
- *Building task*—whether the parent and child use the task to build together or separately. *For this code only*, code response as: 0 = no building, 1 = separate, 2 = separate, then together, 3 = together.

Dyad Ratings

- *Child/parent rhythmicity and coordination*—measures the child/parent smoothness of transitions and movement in the task. It takes into consideration not only verbal coordination, but the involvement of body parts, posture, movement, coordination, and transitions from one action to another.
- *Creativity*—measures the level of creativity the dyad has exhibited with the building block task, which can best be assessed from the end product. Higher scores would be reserved for more sophisticated constructions (i.e., multiple layers, color coordinated, more imaginative) in which the child is able to put a coherent description together. Failure to use at least the majority of the blocks would result in a lesser score.
- *Global quality of interaction*—measures the overall quality of the task. It takes into consideration the level of interaction and working together, the balance of the interaction, the overall level of enjoyment of both the child and parent, and the overall manner in which the parent and child interact with each other through both verbal and nonverbal cues.

CHAPTER FOUR

The Role of Caregiver Commitment in Foster Care

Insights from the This Is My Baby Interview

MARY DOZIER, DAMION GRASSO,
OLIVER LINDHIEM, and ERIN LEWIS

Human infants are born biologically dependent upon their caregivers for survival. Evolution has prepared them to depend upon caregivers for protection from predation, co-regulation of temperature, and nourishment, among other things. In terms of our evolutionary history, having a caregiver fully committed to the infant was critical to survival. In this chapter we conceptualize commitment as a caregiver's motivation to have a permanent relationship with her child. Among most parent–infant dyads, parents become strongly committed to their infants. However, among infants who are cared for by surrogate caregivers, commitment may be more variable and hence more important to consider. There are a number of factors that might affect a surrogate caregiver's commitment, including the perception that the relationship with the child will be permanent, the appeal of the child (e.g., how young the infant is, the child's temperament and behavior), and the caregiver's previous experiences of providing surrogate care. We anticipate that because human beings have evolved in such a way that infants are prepared to have a committed caregiver, having an uncommitted caregiver is experienced as devastating. This chapter will examine child and parent characteristics associated with different levels of caregiver commitment, and will discuss ways in which commitment might affect the child's development.

In one of the child welfare offices we visit, a foster mother came in for an appointment with her caseworker. She was carrying her foster infant under her arm much like a football or a sack of potatoes. As the foster mother carried on her business, it almost seemed as if the bundle she carried was inanimate. Neither her actions nor the actions of the child revealed the more usual characteristics of a human baby. This was so unlike experiences we had with many other foster mothers who were interacting with their babies. For example, one foster mother became very choked up as she talked about her fear that her foster child's biological grandmother would try to adopt the child. She had parented the child since birth and the idea of giving the child up panicked her—she thought of the child as her very own. Two features were fundamentally different between these two foster mothers. The highly committed mother appeared "fiercely" protective of her foster child, and she had a sparkle in her eye for this particular baby—features that did not characterize the mother who carried her foster child like a sack of potatoes. In this chapter, we consider how the notion of commitment might fit into attachment theory, evidence that commitment is critical to an infant's development, and changes in policy and practice that might enhance caregiver commitment.

ATTACHMENT THEORY AND COMMITMENT

Contemporary attachment theory does not present commitment as a salient aspect of the caregiver–child relationship. Nonetheless, the concept of commitment was key to John Bowlby's earliest theorizing about attachment. In 1944, Bowlby published "Forty-Four Juvenile Thieves," the results of a study of adolescent boys who had committed crimes. Bowlby found that a number of the boys who had committed thefts had no one in their lives who was fully committed to their well-being. Many of these children appeared incapable of meaningful human relationships, impressing Bowlby with what he considered the devastating impact of not having a committed caregiver. His work with Robertson and Robertson (e.g., Bowlby, 1951) regarding institutional care reinforced his conviction that having a committed caregiver was integral to children's healthy development. Although the concept of commitment in Bowlby's early work was an impetus for developing attachment theory, much of the empirical work and theoretical writing in recent years has focused on attachment quality (i.e., individual differences in attachment behavior) rather than commitment.

We expect that this move away from considering commitment as critical resulted from finding relatively little variability in commitment among parents in typical caregiving contexts. Instead, the emphasis shifted to attachment quality, in which very important individual differences are found among typically developing children using the Strange Situation procedure. The Strange Situation was developed for assessing the child's expectations of his or her parent's availability when distressed. It has proven to be reliable, to have cross-cultural validity, and to have strong predictive validity (Ainsworth, Blehar, Waters, & Wall, 1978; van IJzendoorn, Dijkstra, & Bus, 1995). Thus, attachment quality emerged as a critical construct and the Strange Situation as a powerful procedure.

Our study of young children in the foster care system has taken us back to the issues of commitment that Bowlby articulated a half century ago. We have found commitment to be a key issue for these children. Perhaps just as critical as infants' expectation of whether their parent will soothe them when they are distressed (reflecting attachment quality) is their expectation of whether they can count on their parent's motivation to maintain a permanent relationship with them.

Primatologists studying attachment among nonhuman primates have described dyadic and triadic functions of the attachment system (e.g., Berman & Kapsalis, 1999). Although human attachment researchers have used these terms to refer to different concepts, we describe them here in the way that primatologists have used them. Dyadic attachment refers to the parent's soothing the infant (such as following a threat), whereas triadic attachment refers to the parent's protecting the infant from a threatening third party. These two functions of the attachment system have been found to be orthogonal (Warfield, personal communication). For example, a low-ranking female may be able to soothe her infant effectively, but not be able to protect the infant from high-ranking troop members, thus effectively soothing (dyadic function) but not protecting (triadic function). Conversely, a dismissing mother may not soothe her infant effectively (dyadic function), but may be quite able and willing to protect her infant from threat (triadic function).

Dyadic attachment, as defined by primatologists, is assessed in the Strange Situation. The child's expectation that the parent will soothe him or her is assessed as the parent and child are reunited following each of two separations. What is not assessed in this procedure is whether the child expects the parent to protect him or her (i.e., the triadic function described by primatologists). This triadic function is most similar to what we are talking about as commitment.

EXAMPLES OF HIGH AND LOW COMMITMENT

Justin went home from the hospital with his foster mother, Ms. Lee, and lived with her continuously for the first 14 months of his life. Watching Justin and Ms. Lee together was a joy. She beamed as he kicked a ball around her living room, and fretted when she was separated from him in the Strange Situation. Justin appeared passionate about Ms. Lee, proudly showing her when he figured out how to put one toy inside another, and excitedly running to her and jumping into her arms when she returned following the Strange Situation separation. He was Ms. Lee's first foster child. Several years earlier, Ms. Lee had decided not to have biological children due to a history of mental illness in her family. Justin, however, had become her child. She thought of him when she spent the day away from home. She sparkled when she talked about how loving Justin had become. She worried that someday a grandparent might show up who wanted to adopt him. Although most birth parents do not have the anxiety that Ms. Lee had about the permanence of the relationship with her children, there was little that separated her and a birth parent in terms of how "fiercely" protective she felt of her child and the "sparkle in her eye" as she talked proudly about her child. It was clear that Ms. Lee felt, as most birth parents do, that "this is my baby."

Larry was also 14 months old. He had been placed in two foster homes prior to his placement with Ms. Duncan, one for a period of 3 months and one for 3 weeks. He had now lived with Ms. Duncan for 6 months. Ms. Duncan had worked as a foster parent for the last two decades and had fostered a total of 46 children. Although she talked emotionally about two of the children she had fostered very early on, she more recently appeared to keep some distance from the children in her care. In addition to Larry, Ms. Duncan currently had three children living with her. A 3-year-old special needs girl was in her care, as was a 28-

month-old boy. Her interactions with Larry were much more difficult to watch than were the interactions between Justin and Ms. Lee. Following their separation in the Strange Situation, Larry partially approached Ms. Duncan, but kept some distance. He appeared worried, seeming eager to get closer. Ms. Duncan did not offer any help to him. As she talked about Larry, it was wholly different than how Ms. Lee talked about her children. She did not think of this child as her own, but rather one that she was caring for. When discussing Larry's developmental changes, the most salient change she noted was the point when he was no longer willing to stay in his car seat, thus requiring more of her time.

There are a number of things that differentiate Justin and Larry, but surely one is the level of commitment that their caregivers have toward them. Having been impressed with this issue at an anecdotal level, we decided to develop an interview that would measure caregiver commitment.

We developed the This Is My Baby (TIMB; Bates & Dozier, 1998) interview, in which parents are asked to talk about their feelings about their child and to respond to questions regarding their relationship with the child. In particular, parents are asked how much they would miss the child if the child were to leave their care, and whether they wished that they could raise the child, among other things (see Appendix 4.1). The TIMB is administered in a semistructured format and then coded. Commitment and two closely related and overlapping factors (Acceptance and Belief in Influence) are measured in the TIMB. Our focus in this chapter is on caregiver commitment, which is quantified using a 5-point Likert scale (1 = lowest commitment, 5 = highest commitment).

The following was taken from Ms. Lee's TIMB transcript.

INTERVIEWER: Would you like to raise Justin?

MS. LEE: Oh, absolutely. That's what I want more than anything. Sometimes I just feel a sense of panic that I wouldn't be able to raise him. It would be horrible for him—and for me!

INTERVIEWER: What would happen if he were removed from your care?

MS. LEE: I feel like I'd leave the state, leave the country. I know that I wouldn't, or shouldn't, but I can't stand the thought of him being placed with someone else. I'm all he knows as a mother. My worker has told me not to count on having him stay with me, but that's nothing that Justin can understand. I guess at some point, it became something that I couldn't understand. He is my baby.

The example above, taken from Ms. Lee's transcript, clearly conveys the idea that Ms. Lee has a strong desire and willingness to parent Justin and that she would miss him deeply if he had to leave her care. The above passages earn Ms. Lee a score of 5 on the 5-point Commitment scale of the TIMB interview because these statements provide strong evidence that Ms. Lee views Justin as her own child, that parenting Justin is an important part of her life, and that Ms. Lee clearly wants her involvement in Justin's life to continue. In order to earn a score of 5, it is necessary for the parent to elaborate his or her responses, as seen is Ms. Lee's transcript, indicating that he or she has thought extensively about these issues regarding *this particular child*. In addition, each TIMB transcript is coded from the audio-recorded interview. Therefore, the tone that the parent uses to respond to these questions is influential in assigning the parent's score. Thus, it is rare for a parent to earn a score of 5 if his or her tone when responding to these questions is flat, lacking the affective component suggesting an investment in this child.

Another example of a response typical of parents scoring a 5 on Commitment is provided below.

INTERVIEWER: How much would you miss Matthew if he had to leave your care?

PARENT: It would actually kill me—, actu—, I mean it would be devastating, it would be the most, I, I can't, I actually couldn't even imagine it. It would be so devastating (*starts to cry*). Oh, my God. It would break my heart. I think that would be like any mother losing their child. It would, it would devastate me. You know, you wonder if you could ever go on.

On the opposite end of the Commitment spectrum, the following was taken from Ms. Duncan's transcript.

INTERVIEWER: Would you like to raise Larry?

MS. DUNCAN: That won't happen. He'll be placed in an adoptive home if his parents can't get it together. He'll turn out to be a good boy, I think, although he won't if he follows in his father's footsteps. I wouldn't know what to do with him when he got to be a teenager. I'm best with babies.

INTERVIEWER: What would happen if he were removed from your care?

MS. DUNCAN: Oh, I think he'll miss me. But I've seen a lot of kids and they adjust. They get used to somebody new. Sometimes it takes a day, sometimes a week, sometimes just an hour. So, he'll be OK. He's not my child, and I never forget that. I never let him forget it either—he tried calling me "mama" sometimes and I always corrected him. "I'd say, "No, I'm Ms. Janie. I'm not your mama." I've seen foster parents get attached to their kids and I think that's just a huge mistake.

In contrast to Ms. Lee's transcript, Ms. Duncan's statements indicate that she does not wish to raise Larry, and in fact she seems to prefer the idea of not raising Larry when he is older. In addition, Ms. Duncan states that she has actively attempted to limit the mother–child bond between herself and Larry. She also shows indifference as to what will happen to Larry when he leaves her care. In listening to Ms. Duncan's interview, these statements were made in a matter-of-fact manner, conveying that Ms. Duncan clearly lacks the emotional investment in parenting Larry that was seen in Ms. Lee's transcript.

The following passage is another example of a parent who was rated a 1 on Commitment.

INTERVIEWER: How much would you miss Charlotte if she had to leave your care?

PARENT: Oh, I'd miss her. I miss all of the children that go because I fall in love with all of them. But, she will be leaving, and I know that when they come into care that they'll all be leaving at some point, so I can't be too upset about it.

These interviews are strikingly different from one another. Ms. Lee is coded at the high end (the "This is my baby" end) of the scale, whereas Ms. Duncan is coded at the low end (the "sack of potatoes" end). As we began to collect interviews from these and other foster mothers, we found that our anecdotal observations of parent–child interactions were borne out by what parents were telling us. That is, parents who treat their children more like "a sack of potatoes" earn very low scores, whereas those who treat their children as birth children earn very high scores on the Commitment scale. Other examples of parents who earned low scores on commitment were those who kept their foster children in a different part of the house than their biological children, and parents who kept their three foster infants in car seats nearly all the time. Examples of high-commitment parents were those who went to great lengths to get permission to take their foster child across state lines for a vacation, and those who celebrated holidays by including their foster children just as they had previously included their birth children.

While the examples drawn from these two transcripts demonstrate the range of different responses we have found in conducting this interview, many parents earn Commitment scores of 2, 3, and 4, responses for which coding is not so clear-cut. The following paragraphs provide further excerpts, taken from TIMB transcripts collected by our lab, in order to show the less extreme responses often given by parents. Brief explanations for how each excerpt was coded are also provided.

A score of 3 on the TIMB is indicative of a moderate level of commitment. This score is assigned when a parent's response is "average." That is, these scores are given when a parent's statements are in line with what an emotionally invested parent would say, but the degree of elaboration in the response is limited and the parent's tone is less warm and less believable than that of a parent earning a higher score on the scale. In these transcripts, parents often say the "right thing," thereby preventing them from earning lower scores, but their responses are less believable than those of highly committed parents.

The following is an excerpt taken from a transcript receiving a score of 3.

INTERVIEWER: Do you ever wish you could raise Meghan?

PARENT: Oh, of course, yes.

INTERVIEWER: And how much would you miss her if she had to leave?

PARENT: Um, I'd miss her a lot. Um, a lot. Yeah. I mean it's been over a
    year that I've had her.

The lack of elaboration in this response provides limited evidence that the parent has ever thought about these issues before, suggesting that these questions, and this child, are not as important to this particular parent as they would be to a highly committed parent. A score of 3 would also be assigned if the evidence for the parent's emotional investment was mixed, with the parent expressing some indicators of high commitment to the child but also some indicators of low commitment.

A score of 4 on the Commitment scale is assigned when a parent provides more evidence, or more compelling evidence, than a parent scoring a 3, but the parent's responses are not as elaborated on or affectively charged as a parent scoring a 5.

For example, the answers of a parent scoring a 4 on Commitment are provided below.

INTERVIEWER: Do you ever wish you could raise Sean?

PARENT: Yes.

INTERVIEWER: And how much would you miss Sean if he had to leave?

PARENT: A whole lot 'cause he's attached to me, and I'm attached to him now. My mom's attached to him. Everybody in my family—my boyfriend's attached to him. So, you know, it would hurt.

A score of 2 on Commitment is assigned when the evidence of a parent's emotional investment in raising the child and wanting the relationship to continue is weak, but there is some evidence. Parents receiving this score are not very convincing in their responses to the interview questions, but they are not indifferent about the child staying in their care, and they do not actually wish the child to be removed from their care. They also provide some evidence of being attached to the child, unlike parents receiving scores of 1.

The following example was taken from a transcript of a parent scoring a 2 on the Commitment scale.

INTERVIEWER: Do you ever wish you could raise Michael?

PARENT: I have, but you know, I couldn't. I think he's really going to be a handful and, given my age, I don't think I could really handle that again. I've thought about it, but I don't think I could.

INTERVIEWER: How much would you miss him if he had to leave?

PARENT: Oh, I think I'd miss him. Um, I don't think it's at the point where I would say I couldn't see him leave, but I, we, would miss him. We had to go someplace in July and he went to respite for two days and we, we did miss him. It was really strange, you know, like he's not here.

One of the issues that we had worried about was the role that social desirability played in the reporting of commitment. However, whereas many self-report measures are problematic in terms of social desirability, our observations had suggested that assessing commitment through self-report would be less susceptible to social desirability biases. Indeed, many parents felt that they had become committed to their foster children *even though* they had been warned against becoming committed by agency staff. Thus, highly committed foster parents often seemed somewhat chagrined over their high level of commitment.

We have found that separate coders can rate commitment on the TIMB reliably. Interrater reliability was calculated as a Pearson correlation and has averaged .90 for commitment as measured by the TIMB (Ackerman & Dozier, 2005). In addition, parents' reports of commitment are relatively stable across time. Test–retest reliability over an 11-month period is $r = .61$ at $p < .01$ (Lindhiem & Dozier, in press). We reasoned that the best test of the TIMB's validity would be its ability to predict whether the relationship endured or disrupted over time. To assess this, we examined commitment as a predictor of relationship stability over a 2-year period (Dozier & Lindhiem, in press). Children were almost twice as likely to be in placement for 2 years or longer for each point increase in caregiver commitment (odds ratio of 1.812). For example, a foster mother who scored a 4 on commitment was almost twice as likely to have her child in placement for 2 years or longer as a foster mother who scored a 3 on commitment. There are surely reasons other than commitment that children are moved, including the birth parent being deemed appropriate to parent, or a relative emerging as a possible foster or adoptive parent. Nonetheless, we had expected and found that the extent to which caregivers feel committed to children is at least one of the variables affecting whether the relationship remains stable.

ASSOCIATIONS BETWEEN COMMITMENT AND OTHER VARIABLES

As we thought through the important variables that we expected would differentiate parents who became more committed from those with lower commitment levels, several characteristics of the parent and of the child seemed salient. We expected that specific aspects of parents and children would predict foster parents' commitment to their child.

Parents who had fostered multiple children were less likely to commit to a new child placed in their care compared to parents who had not fostered many children. Indeed, some parents had fostered more than 100 children, whereas others were fostering their first child. Foster parents are often told that their relationship with the child is only temporary and that they must expect the child's eventual departure with no legal authority in deciding what is in the child's best interest. As expected, we found that the number of children a parent had previously fostered predicted her commitment to her current foster child on the TIMB (Dozier & Lindhiem, in press).

Child characteristics that seemed likely to be important included the age at which children were placed into care and the degree to which children showed behavior problems. Age at placement was expected to be important for a variety of reasons. First, the young of many species have a number of characteristics that are perceived as "cute" and have been proposed as evolving so as to elicit caregiving behaviors (Lorenz, 1942). For example, babies' large foreheads, large, round eyes, and small, round noses are characteristics that are considered cute by many adults (Fullard & Reiling, 1976; Lorenz, 1942). Children gradually lose these babylike characteristics, however, and we thus expected caregivers to show less commitment to children placed at later ages. In a related vein, characteristics of babies, such as the full dependence of a young baby, were expected to elicit more commitment than elicited from older babies. As predicted, we found that the age at which children were placed in care was associated with the level of commitment parents showed. More specifically, parents were rated as more committed to children who were placed at younger versus older ages (Dozier & Lindhiem, in press).

We also expected the level of children's behavior problems to affect caregivers' level of commitment. Especially among older children, we expected that children with more serious behavior problems would have parents who were less committed to them than parents of children with fewer behavior problems. Indeed, we found that the level of child behavior problems reported by foster mothers was associated with the level of caregiver commitment as measured by the TIMB, with greater commitment associated with lower behavior problems (Lindhiem & Dozier, in press). These analyses did not indicate the direction of causality, however, with it being just as plausible that behavior affected commitment, that commitment affected behavior, or that some third variable caused both.

We did not have clear hypotheses regarding associations between attachment state of mind and commitment. As discussed above, we consider the constructs of attachment and commitment relatively orthogonal. In general, among birth mothers, we expect that dismissing mothers would be as likely as other mothers to feel a strong sense of protectiveness regarding their child, even though they might not feel comfortable providing nurturance. This would argue for no association between commitment and attachment state of mind. On the other hand, it might be more difficult for autonomous mothers than others to maintain a low sense of commitment to a child. Our results to date suggest that commitment and attachment state of mind are only weakly associated at most. The primary difference seen is that autonomous mothers do not continue to foster many children over time, whereas dismissing mothers sometimes do. When controlling for number of children fostered, no association between attachment state of mind and commitment is seen.

WHY COMMITMENT IS IMPORTANT

Humans have evolved in such a way that the human infant is totally dependent on the caregiver at birth. Unlike the newly hatched sea turtle who must make the long crawl from the nest in the sand to the ocean alone to survive, and even the rhesus who can cling to the mother from birth, the human infant is fully dependent on the parent to hold, carry, and provide sustenance. The human infant has systems in place to elicit caregiving nonetheless. Already mentioned are characteristics that are considered cute, such as large forehead, round eyes, and rounded nose. Also, the infant's preference for gazing into the parent's eyes and the rooting reflex serve as very effective elicitors of care (Blauvelt, 1962). Evolution has also prepared parents for caregiving. The hormones produced at high levels in childbirth and lactation, especially oxytocin, appear important in regulating caregiving (Pedersen, 1997). Oxytocin is produced in higher quantities than usual during pregnancy and lactation (Carter & Altemus, 1997; Carter et al., 1997). Higher levels of oxytocin are associated with more responsive caregiving (Pedersen, 1997) and with global changes that may facilitate caregiving, including greater calmness and tolerance for both stress and monotony (Carter & Altemus, 1997; Levine, 1983).

Thus, babies are evolutionarily prepared to have committed parents, and parents (especially mothers) are evolutionarily prepared to commit to their child. We suggest that there could be nothing more threatening for a baby than not having a committed caregiver. Having a committed caregiver may be more essential than having a soothing caregiver, and more urgent than even having physical needs met. The child that lacks a committed caregiver is vulnerable to a range of threats. For example, a noncommitted parent might not be willing to sacrifice in order to protect the child from danger. Thus, the child who lacks a committed caregiver likely experiences an urgent, but chronic, state of alarm. We expect that not having a committed caregiver leads to children adapting in ways that have problematic long-term effects on neurobiology and behavior.

We have found that a caregiver's level of commitment predicts how long a foster child remains in placement with the caregiver, reflecting the stability of the placement and the relationship (Dozier & Lindhiem, in press). Stability in care has been found to be a powerful predictor of long-term outcomes for foster children. For example, foster children who experience multiple placements are likely to experience academic difficulties (Aldgate, Colton, Ghate, & Heath, 1992) and to have elevated levels of behavior problems (Fisher, Burraston, & Pears, 2005). In the United States approximately 17% of children in 2001 had three or more placements in their first year in care (U.S. Department of Health and Human Services, 2003). In smaller-scale studies, this proportion is much higher, with some children changing placements as many as five times in 1 year (DeSena et al., 2005; Newton, Litrownik, & Landsverk, 2000; Rubin, Alessandrini, Feudtner, Localio, & Hadley, 2004; Webster, Barth, & Needell, 2000). Thus, the public health significance of having a committed foster parent seems impressive.

CLINICAL IMPLICATIONS

The foster care system was designed to provide temporary care for children. Low levels of caregiver commitment are inherent in such a system. Until relatively recently, the foster care and adoption systems were not integrated. Foster parents were often not licensed as adoptive parents and vice versa. Foster parents were not encouraged to attempt to adopt children, partly because doing so would deplete the supply of foster parents willing to take children into their homes on a temporary basis. Instead, clinicians and caseworkers often cautioned foster parents not to become too "attached" to the children in their care. In 2001, a total of 126,000 children whose biological parents' rights were terminated had been waiting to be adopted for more than 5 years. Of the 46,668 foster children adopted in 2001, about half were adopted by their foster parents. The remaining 113,380 foster children continued to wait for permanent caregivers (U.S. Department of Health and Human Services,

2003). Although various federal and state programs strive to increase incentives to adopt, the recruitment and training of foster parents still often takes place without adoption in mind, especially when reunification is the initial goal. Foster parents caring for children with reunification as a goal often have not discussed with caseworkers the feasibility of adopting the child should reunification efforts fail. Too often, foster care provides only temporary solutions to critical situations. We have more work to do in order to fully understand caregiver commitment. Nonetheless, given what we know at this point, we suggest several possible strategies that might enhance foster parents' commitment for the children in their care.

1. *Provide services to birth parents prior to disrupting the relationship.* If reunification is considered likely, we suggest the importance of clinicians and caseworkers working intensively with mother and child together rather than separating the dyad. One example of outstanding work is being conducted by Jude Cassidy, in collaboration with Bert Powell, Kent Hoffman, Glen Cooper, and Robert Marvin. Whereas mothers who are imprisoned are routinely separated from their infants, Cassidy and colleagues set up a Baltimore prison such that mothers were randomly assigned to conditions as usual or were housed with their babies. The mothers with their babies were given the "Circle of Security" intervention (see Powell et al., Chapter 7, this volume). The interventionists described mothers as highly motivated for the intervention partly because other activities were restricted, thus providing an excellent environment for learning (J. Cassidy, personal communication). This structure (i.e., housing mothers and babies together and providing services) makes an enormous amount of sense as the default strategy.

When foster children themselves have babies, it is becoming more common to keep the adolescent girl and her child together in a foster home. Foster mothers can support the girls in their growth as mothers, and can model appropriate caregiving. Foster mothers also provide appropriate care to the infant where it is lacking. Ideally, the foster parents would establish an enduring and permanent relationship with the adolescent girl and her child so as to establish themselves as a continuing resource and positive support.

2. *Create conditions that favor foster parent commitment.* Only when reunification is thought to be unlikely do we suggest that young children be placed in foster care. For babies, especially, we suggest that these be prospective adoptive homes whenever possible. This practice

involves the dual licensing of foster and adoptive families, making it easier for foster parents to adopt the children in their care (Wulczyn, Hislop, & Harden, 2002). Furthermore, changing the system such that clinicians and caseworkers encourage foster parents to remain in children's lives over time (even when returning to birth parent homes) would allow foster parents to commit in ways that are not as likely otherwise. For example, creating a system in which foster parents support birth parents and remain in children's lives as "godparents" or aunts and uncles would allow them to psychologically commit even when permanent placement is not likely.

3. *Provide foster parents with specialized training and support.* When infants are placed into foster care after 10 to 12 months of age, they behave in ways that make it more difficult for foster parents to behave in nurturing ways than when they are placed at younger ages (Stovall & Dozier, 2000; Stovall-McClough & Dozier, 2004). Older infants tend to behave in avoidant or resistant ways when distressed, which communicates to parents that they are not needed or that the parents are not adequate to take care of their needs. Caregivers tend to respond "in kind," to infants' signals, responding as if their infants do not need them, or even responding angrily. Foster infants and toddlers who exhibit difficult behaviors are at increased risk for placement disruptions. We have developed an intervention, Attachment and Biobehavioral Catch-up, that targets several key issues including the provision of nurturance for distressed infants even when parents are not comfortable providing nurturance, overriding tendencies to respond "in kind" to infant behaviors and providing a predictable interpersonal environment for the infant. It is our hope that this intervention will equip clinicians and caseworkers with techniques to train foster parents to care for young foster children in ways that facilitate stable and nurturing home environments.

CONCLUSION

More work is needed in order to fully understand the role of caregiver commitment in young children's healthy development and functioning and to promote ways to enhance commitment in foster care. We know that caregiver commitment is related to certain child characteristics (e.g., behavior problems and age at placement) and caregiver characteristics (e.g., previous foster parenting experience) and that it is associated with important outcomes for foster children (e.g., placement stability). Changing the system such that foster parents can expect to remain in children's lives over time, even after reunification, would allow foster parents to commit in ways that are not as likely otherwise. By acting in ways that might promote caregiver commitment, we expect to improve opportunities for foster children to establish long-lasting relationships with primary caregivers and go on to attain positive outcomes, perhaps "beating the odds."

REFERENCES

Ackerman, J. P., & Dozier, M. (2005). The influence of foster parent investment on children's representations of self and attachment figures. *Journal of Applied Developmental Psychology, 26*(5), 507–520.

Ainsworth, M. S., Blehar, M. C., Waters, E., & Wall, S. (1978). *Patterns of attachment: A psychological study of the Strange Situation.* Oxford, UK: Erlbaum.

Aldgate, J., Colton, M., Ghate, D., & Heath, A. (1992). Educational attainment and stability in long-term foster care. *Children and Society, 6*(2), 91–103.

Bates, B., & Dozier, M. (1998). *"This Is My Baby" coding manual.* Unpublished manuscript, University of Delaware, Newark.

Berman, C. M., & Kapsalis, E. (1999). Development of kin bias among rhesus monkeys: Maternal transmission or individual learning? *Animal Behavior, 58,* 883–894.

Blauvelt, H. H. (1962). Capacity of a human neonate reflex to signal future response by present action. *Child Development, 33*(1), 21–28.

Bowlby, J. (1944). Forty-four juvenile thieves: Their characters and home-life. *International Journal of Psycho-Analysis, 25,* 19–53.

Bowlby, J. (1951). *Maternal care and mental health.* Geneva, Switzerland: World Health Organization.

Carter, C. S., & Altemus, M. (1997). Integrative functions of lactational hormones in social behavior and stress management. *Annals of the New York Academy of Sciences, 807,* 164–174.

Carter, C. S., DeVries, A. C., Taymans, S. E., Roberts, R. L., Williams, J. R., & Getz, L. L. (1997). Peptides, steroids, and pair bonding. *Annals of the New York Academy of Sciences, 807,* 260–272.

DeSena, A. D., Murphy, R. A., Douglas-Palumberi, H., Blau, G., Kelly, B., Horwitz, S. M., et al. (2005). SAFE Homes: Is it worth the cost? An evaluation of a group home permanency planning program for children who first enter out-of-home care. *Child Abuse and Neglect, 29,* 627–643.

Dozier, M., & Lindhiem, O. (in press). This is my child: Differences among foster parents in commitment to their young children. *Child Maltreatment.*

Fisher, P. A., Burraston, B., & Pears, K. (2005). The Early Intervention Foster Care Program: Permanent placement outcomes from a randomized trial.

Child Maltreatment: Journal of the American Professional Society on the Abuse of Children, 10(1), 61–71.

Fullard, W., & Reiling, A. M. (1976). An investigation of Lorenz's "babyness." *Child Development, 47*(4), 1191–1193.

Levine, S. (1983). A psychobiological approach to the ontogeny of coping. In N. Garmezy & M. Rutter (Eds.), *Stress, coping and development in children* (pp. 107–131). New York: McGraw-Hill.

Lindhiem, O., & Dozier, M. (in press). Caregiver commitment to foster children: The role of child characteristics. *Child Abuse and Neglect.*

Lorenz, K. (1942). The innate conditions of the possibility of experience. *Zietschrift für Tierpsychologie, 5,* 235–409.

Newton, R. R., Litrownik, A. J., & Landsverk, J. A. (2000). Children and youth in foster care: Distangling the relationship between problem behaviors and number of placements. *Child Abuse and Neglect, 24*(10), 1363–1374.

Pedersen, C. A. (1997). Oxytocin control of maternal behavior: Regulation by sex steroids and offspring stimuli. *Annals of the New York Academy of Sciences, 807,* 126–145.

Rubin, D. M., Alessandrini, E. A., Feudtner, C., Localio, A. R., & Hadley, T. (2004). Placement changes and emergency department visits in the first year of foster care. *Pediatrics, 114*(3), e354–e360.

Stovall, K. C., & Dozier, M. (2000). The development of attachment in new relationships: Single subject analyses for 10 foster infants. *Development and Psychopathology, 12*(2), 133–156.

Stovall-McClough, K. C., & Dozier, M. (2004). Forming attachments in foster care: Infant attachment behaviors during the first 2 months of placement. *Development and Psychopathology, 16*(2), 253–271.

U.S. Department of Health and Human Services, Administration on Children, Youth and Families. (2003). *Child welfare outcomes 2001: Annual report.* Washington, DC: U.S. Government Printing Office.

van IJzendoorn, M. H., Dijkstra, J., & Bus, A. G. (1995). Attachment, intelligence, and language: A meta-analysis. *Social Development, 4*(2), 115–128.

Webster, D., Barth, R. P., & Needell, B. (2000). Placement stability for children in out-of-home care: a longitudinal analysis. *Child Welfare, 79*(5), 614–632.

Wulczyn, F., Hislop, K. B., & Harden, B. J. (2002). The placement of infants in foster care. *Infant Mental Health Journal, 23*(5), 454–475.

Appendix 4.1. This Is My Baby (TIMB)
Interview Questions and Rating Guidelines

TIMB Interview Questions

1. I would like to begin by asking you to describe (child's name). What is (his/her) personality like?
2. Do you ever wish you could raise (child's name)?
3. How much would you miss (child's name) if (he/she) had to leave?
4. How do you think your relationship with (child's name) is affecting (him/her) right now?
5. How do you think your relationship with (child's name) will affect (him/her) in the long term?
6. What do you want for (child's name) right now?
7. What do you want for (child's name) in the future?
8. Is there anything about (child's name) or your relationship that we've not touched on that you'd like to tell me?
9. I'd like to end by asking a few basic questions about your experience as a foster parent:
   a. How long have you been a foster parent?
   b. How many foster children have you cared for in all?
   c. How many foster children do you currently have?
   d. How many biological and/or adopted children are currently living in your home?

TIMB Commitment Ratings

- *5 points (high commitment):* The mother provides evidence of a strong emotional investment in the child and in parenting the child; multiple indices of high levels of commitment are present throughout the interview; descriptions of the child and the mother–child relationship clearly reflect a strong attachment to the child with no evidence of mental or physical activities designed to limit the strength of the mother–child affective bond; there is evidence of the mother committing resources to promote the child's growth, or other indices of psychological adoption of the child; the child is fully integrated into the family; although the mother may acknowledge that the child will eventually leave her home (e.g., to return to the biological parent) she considers the child as hers while the child is in her home.

- *3 points (moderate commitment):* The mother provides evidence of investment in the child, but this is not clearly as marked as a mother scoring high on commitment; although there may be some indices of high levels of commitment, there may also be evidence suggesting that the child has not been psychologically adopted by the mother; the mother may state she would miss the child if he or she left, but this is more of a matter-of-fact statement and lacks the strong affective component seen in mothers high in commitment; if the mother speaks of limiting the psychological bond with the infant, she also gives evidence of struggling with this issue; the child may be only partially integrated into the family (i.e., is placed in respite care only when the family goes on vacation); overall, the coder may conclude that the child is adequately care for and nurtured, but not to any special degree.

- *1 point (low commitment):* The mother provides virtually no evidence of a strong and active emotional investment in the child or in parenting the child; there are few, if any, indices of high levels of commitment; the mother may be indifferent to whether the child remains in her care or may actually state that she hopes/desires that the child will be removed; there may be little evidence that the mother would miss the child if he or she leaves; the mother may provide evidence of participating in physical or mental activities designed to limit the strength of the mother–child bond; the child has not been psychologically adopted by the mother, and may not be fully integrated into the family (e.g., is routinely placed in respite care); the child may seem to be more of an unwelcome guest than a member of the family, or may be viewed as only one of a series of children passing through the mother's home.

CHAPTER FIVE

Parental Resolution of the Child's Diagnosis and the Parent–Child Relationship

Insights from the Reaction to Diagnosis Interview

DAVID OPPENHEIM, SMADAR DOLEV,
NINA KOREN-KARIE, EFRAT SHER-CENSOR,
NURIT YIRMIYA, and SHAHAF SALOMON

Most parents who receive a diagnosis of a serious developmental disorder like autism for their child experience strong emotional reactions such as shock, sadness, despair, or confusion. Many have likened this experience to a metaphorical loss of the child: It is as if the wished-for, typically developing child has been lost, and instead parents are faced with many questions, anxieties, and fears regarding their child's development. From the perspective of attachment theory, parents who successfully cope with the emotions evoked by their child's diagnosis and who, over time, revise their view of the child, are considered "resolved" with respect to the diagnosis. Resolution is thought to foster acceptance of the child and to promote caregiving that is matched to the child's unique characteristics. Consequently, resolution is likely to contribute to children's sense of being understood, accepted, and secure. Parental lack of resolution, on the other hand, involves difficulties in revising the view of the child in light of the diagnosis, and can therefore lead to responses that are not congruent with the child's needs. Clinicians working with parents of children who receive diagnoses can play an important role in facilitating the resolution process, with likely positive effects for both parents and children. The goals of this chapter are to introduce both the concept of resolution and vignettes that illustrate how resolution (and lack thereof) is reflected in parental interviews. In addition we summarize research findings linking resolution status to parental and child characteristics as well as to parent–child interactions. We end with a discussion regarding the implications of this research for clinical work with parents.

As the point of departure of our theoretical discussion, we consider the emotional experience of receiving a diagnosis as a loss, and we therefore begin by presenting Bowlby's original formulations about loss and mourning.

LOSS AND MOURNING: BOWLBY'S THEORY

Based on research on bereaved individuals as well as on clinical experience, Bowlby described four phases that generally characterize the process of mourning: Numbing, yearning and searching for the lost figure, disorganization and despair, and "greater or lesser" reorganization (Bowlby, 1980). Bowlby considered this sequence as generally characteristic but acknowledged many individual variations, with possible oscillations from phase to phase, as well as overlaps between phases. Bowlby described *reorganization* as the optimal and healthy outcome of mourning, involving alignment of the person's representational world in line with the new reality that includes the loss. Such alignment includes accepting the irreversible nature of the loss, working through and discarding old patterns of thinking, feeling, and acting, and a gradual acceptance that the loss is in truth permanent, and that life has to be shaped anew. Although this process is suffused with a wide spectrum of heightened and intense emotions, the process is not only affective and does not only involve the discharge of painful affects. For Bowlby, the cognitive reshaping of internal working models and the redefinition of the self and others are a sine qua non for a healthy mourning process. It is this reshaping that will enable the grieving person to adapt to the new reality and to the life circumstances following the loss. Conversely, failing to reshape working models in line with the loss limits the capacity of the individual to adapt, because the internal models and the external reality are incongruent.

In this chapter we discuss similar reshaping of the internal working models of parents whose child has received a severe developmental diagnosis such as autism spectrum disorder. Parents need to realign their working models of the child in light of the diagnosis, and this realignment is likely to promote caregiving that is congruent with the child's needs. Studies of this process have relied on attachment research on the resolution of loss and trauma, and we review this literature next.

RESOLUTION OF LOSS OR TRAUMA: MAIN AND HESSE

Attachment research on the resolution of loss and trauma has primarily been retrospective. Main and Hesse (1990) studied the reorganization of the representational world by examining the outcome of the mourning process using interviews of individuals regarding their past experiences of loss. To assess individuals' states of mind regarding their past, Main and Hesse used the Adult Attachment Interview (AAI; Main, Kaplan, & Cassidy, 1985), in which adults are asked about their childhood attachment experiences, including experiences of loss. The AAI is used to classify adults' general state of mind with respect to their attachment history. More pertinent here is the classification of interviewees' mental states as *resolved* or *unresolved* with respect to past losses and/or traumas. For Main and Hesse lapses in monitoring of speech or thought while discussing losses or traumas indicate lack of resolution. The lapses, such as shifting to speech in the present tense when describing the trauma, or talking about deceased persons as if they were alive, are thought to indicate the failure to integrate the loss experience into the representational system and to realign working models with a new reality that includes the loss. Thus, from this perspective a resolved state of mind is equivalent to the reorganization phase in Bowlby's scheme, although interestingly, Bowlby himself did not use the term *resolution*.

For Main and Hesse lack of resolution is important because of its implications for parenting and, in turn, the child's attachment. The central focus of their work was to identify the way parents' states of mind regarding their past, and in particular regarding past losses and traumas, predict the attachment status of their children. Main and Hesse argued that lack of resolution can interfere with parenting because it interferes with the accurate reading of the child's signals: Parents who are unresolved are likely to be distressed or frightened in attachment caregiving interactions, and will either (1) display caregiving that is incomprehensible and frightening to the child, (2) communicate to the child that he or she is a source of alarm, perhaps because they confuse the child with their attachment figures, or (3) avoid the child when attachment needs are heightened (Lyons-Ruth & Spielman, 2004; Main & Hesse, 1990; Marvin & Pianta, 1996). The child, in turn, may surmise that his or her attachment behaviors and needs frighten the parent, or lead the parent to frightening behavior. Thus, being unresolved with regard to loss interferes with the parent's capacity to accurately read the child's signals and respond appropriately, increasing the chances that an insecure and, particularly, disorganized attachment between the child and the parent will develop. Numerous studies support this hypothesis and reveal that unresolved status of the parent is associated with disorganized attachment between the child and the parent (van IJzendoorn, Schuengel, & Bakermans-Kranenburg, 1999).

If lack of resolution of past loss or trauma disrupts parenting and is associated with insecure/disorganized attachment, will a similar outcome be evident when parents fail to resolve the experience of receiving a diagnosis for their child? This question guided the research of Pianta and Marvin to which we turn next.

RESOLUTION WITH RESPECT TO A DIAGNOSIS FOR THE CHILD: PIANTA AND MARVIN

Pianta and Marvin (Marvin & Pianta, 1996; Pianta, Marvin, Britner, & Borowitz, 1996; Pianta, Marvin, & Morog, 1999) studied parents of children who received diagnoses of cerebral palsy or epilepsy and, like others, conceptualized their experience as a loss that triggers an emotionally painful process that shares many similarities with grief and mourning. The parents' reactions were studied retrospectively by interviewing them months, and more often years, after the diagnosis had been given. In fact, by definition, issues of resolution can *only* be examined after a considerable time has passed since the parents received the diagnosis. Pianta and Marvin define resolution as the "integration of the experience of the diagnosis into the parent's representations which allows for a reorientation and refocus of attention and problem solving on present reality." Thus they adopted Bowlby's emphasis on successful adjustment to a loss as involving realignment of working models. Such realignment enables the parent to both recognize and accept the child's diagnosis and to see the uniqueness and individuality of the child beyond the diagnosis. Pianta and Marvin argued that lack of such realignment becomes a barrier for caregiving. Parents may interact with the child as if he or she were the wished-for, typically developing child, effectively denying the child's difficulties. Or, they may see the child only through the prism of the diagnosis, ignoring other aspects of the child's personality. Other parents are overwhelmed with grief, and still others may focus on the failures of professionals. As will be described below, the lack of resolution can be expressed in many ways, but all have in common the parents' difficulty focusing their attention and resources on the present reality of the child and the child's unique needs.

Reaction to Diagnosis Interview

To examine parental resolution Pianta and Marvin developed the Reaction to Diagnosis Interview (RDI; Pianta & Marvin, 1992). The RDI includes five questions in which parents are asked to describe their feelings and thoughts about their child's diagnosis. In the first question parents are asked to describe when they began to notice their child's difficulty, how old the child was at that time, and what were the difficulties that they noticed. This question helps parents focus on their initial thoughts and concerns about their child's difficulties, even before a formal diagnosis has been given. Furthermore, it provides important information regarding the specific story of each family, and the diagnostic process that the child and the family underwent. The second question refers to parents' feelings about their child's difficulty. Here parents are asked to describe their responses to noticing the adverse course their child's development has taken. In the third question parents are asked to describe in detail their feelings, thoughts, and actions surrounding the time that they received the child's diagnosis. This question, which takes many parents back to a very difficult period in their lives, tries to capture their response to the diagnosis immediately after it was given. Parents are asked to describe how they felt, what they thought and did, how this new knowledge affected their lives, and/or what they did to help their child and themselves. The fourth question is the "change" question, in which parents are asked about the changes in their feelings from the day of getting the diagnosis until the present. Finally, in the fifth question, parents are asked about their thoughts as to the reason/s that their child has the specific diagnosis. This provides parents with the opportunity to speak about various ideas that they have regarding the etiology of their child's condition, and regarding existential issues such as why this adversity befell them.

PARENTAL INTERVIEWS REGARDING THE DIAGNOSIS OF AUTISM SPECTRUM DISORDER

In this section we provide examples from our studies of parent–child relationships and parental resolution among families of children diagnosed with autistic disorder or pervasive developmental disorder not otherwise specified (PDD NOS). The first, "preschooler" study (Dolev, 2005) included preschool-age boys between the ages of 2.5 and 5.5 years and their mothers, whereas the second, "family" study (Salomon et al., 2006) included a wider age range of children (mean age around 8 years) and included boys and girls as well as mothers and fathers. This second study is still ongoing, and only partial data regarding 38 children and their parents are available.

The examples are organized around the RDI classification system (Pianta & Marvin, 1993), beginning with illustrations of the resolved classification followed by the unresolved classification. An important goal of the vignettes is to demonstrate the range of styles *within* each classification (i.e., within the resolved and within the unresolved classifications), because both resolution and lack thereof may be expressed in multiple ways that may appear different on the surface but reflect similar underlying organization.

Resolved with Respect to the Child's Diagnosis

Three central features characterize parents who are classified as resolved: (1) the capacity to describe the changes they went through from the time of receiving the diagnosis until the present; (2) acceptance of the child's condition while maintaining hope for improvement; and (3) suspension and lack of preoccupation with the search for a reason and cause for their child's developmental disability. These features will be described first. In addition, the resolved classification is divided into three subclas-sifications reflecting three orientations—thinking, feeling, and action—and they will be described subsequently.

Awareness of Change from the Time of the Diagnosis until the Present

This feature involves parents' description of changes in their feelings, thoughts, and actions surrounding their child's diagnosis and treatment. One mother described vividly the changes she went through during the 2 years that passed from the time she received her child's diagnosis:

> "It took us some time, we had to get over the initial shock. At first all we saw was the autism, the child was—autistic! But as time went by we realized that that wasn't true, he was first of all our child, a wonderful child—he is loving, he is fun, sometimes he is even very funny. Today we are much more focused on doing what is best for him, on helping him. Seeing him work so hard and seeing his prog-ress gives us a lot of strength. The shock and despair are not there any more even though we do worry from time to time, but we also feel a lot of hope."

This mother talks about the change she went through regarding her child's diagnosis—from seeing him primarily through the lens of the autism diagnosis to realizing he was still her child, and that he had many positive characteristics aside from his autism. The changes in her view of her child were accompanied by changes in her feelings—the shock and despair she felt at first changed to a more balanced set of feelings.

Many resolved parents, like this mother, talk about interrelated pro-cesses in which the progress of the child helps them see positive aspects in their child and in their parenting, be more optimistic, and find in them-selves resources for dealing with the present and future. It is important to point out that while the progress these parents describe is believable and seems to be "real," it may represent steps that "objectively" speaking may be rather small. All the children who are described in these interviews were still within the boundaries of the autism/PDD diagnosis at the time of the interview. Thus, what characterizes parents classified as resolved is the change in perspective from the initial diagnosis to the present and their capacity to use developmental gains as hopeful signs for the future.

Acceptance

Resolution also involves acceptance of the child's condition and the reality of living with a child with a significant developmental disorder while maintaining hope for improvement and not despairing. For example, in response to the "change" question, one mother said:

> "Once I thought that the problem will just go away, that he will grow out of it. I thought that we will treat the problem and he will be completely normal, but today I know that it's here to stay. Still, we are working very hard and I believe that in a few years when he will start school he will attend a regular class, although he will probably need some individualized assistance."

This mother speaks about a change in her perception of her child's condition from great difficulties in accepting the reality of the diagnosis with all its implications to a more balanced position. On the one hand, she accepts that her child's disability is permanent and will be part of his life forever, and on the other hand, she shows optimistic (and yet not unrealistic) hope for progress in his functioning.

Some parents evidence their resolved state of mind by speaking about their life as returning to a normal course, and seeing their children as having a range of characteristics and attributes, many of which can be positive and "normal." Most importantly they see the child beyond the diagnostic label. One such mother described this as follows:

> "Today I'm in a completely different place. Surprisingly, life is back to normal, we got on with our lives. You can see his autistic behavior in specific moments, but other than that he is part of our family. I speak to him in the same way that I speak to his brothers. If I ask him to do something, he does it."

It is important to emphasize that resolution, particularly for parents who discuss their feelings during the interview, does not imply that the pain and sadness are no longer present. Some parents still experience these feelings and other negative emotions in the present, but these negative emotions do not overwhelm them. Rather they are part of a wider spectrum of emotions that describes their current state of mind. For example, in response to the "change" question, one mother said:

"From time to time I cry, and worry what will be in his and our future, how will we cope, but these moments are rare. By and large I feel I'm in a different place today. He has progressed so much, and that leaves us full of hope."

Most resolved parents, similar to the mother in the last example, describe positive changes in their thoughts and feelings. Some parents portray negative changes, however. Usually these are parents of older children, who report that their child's functioning did not improve significantly or even deteriorated over the years. They describe a change from optimism and hope to an acceptance of their child's condition. They, too, are considered resolved because of their acceptance of the child as well as their ability to describe authentically and in a contained manner the changes in their thoughts and feelings. For example, in response to the "change" question one father said:

"I think that what changed was that the younger she was, the more hopeful we were. Although we knew she had a problem, and we had some fears, we hoped that if we work hard, there will be an improvement. Let's say we had 20% fear and 80% hope. But as the years passed, as she got older, the pessimistic parts increased, 20% became 30% and then 40% and so on. But at a certain age it ended. We realized that this is our daughter; on the autism scale her condition is quite severe. There are limits to her ability, and she is probably going to stay in this condition for the rest of her life. We keep on going with her to treatments, but we are doing this mainly because we see that it makes her happy. We are realistic and know that we can expect only minor progress."

Suspending the Search for Reasons

The third characteristic of resolved parents is their suspension of the search for the causes for their child's developmental disability. Suspending the search does not mean ceasing to seek information about the disorder or treatment options, but rather not being *preoccupied* by this search. When asked about the causes for their child's disability many of them share their ideas about the causes of their child's disorder. These may include "God's will," genetic factors, or a vaccination the child received. The crucial point in designating these parents as resolved is their acknowledgment that these are only speculations, and that they are not heavily invested in the search for reasons or causes. It seems that in their ongoing, day-to-day life, these parents do not focus on these issues. Thus one mother said, "Maybe it's all from God, but I don't question it so much," and another remarked, "Maybe it's genetic or maybe it's the vaccination he received as a baby . . . there are so many possibilities, you can't really get an answer, so I stopped looking for one."

Suspending the search for causes for the child's difficulties in the present does not mean that parents did not go through a period in which such a search was central, but rather that they are currently not at that point. For example, one father responded to the question about the causes for the child's condition by saying:

> "When we discovered that he has PDD we immediately started thinking what was wrong with us, what could have been wrong in general, and who to blame, because you always look for someone to blame. But later on I started thinking that there is no point in thinking like that. So many things could have caused it, I just don't know. So I decided that instead of spending so much energy in looking for whom to blame, we should invest it in what is more important—in treating our child."

Some parents may even talk about questions that remain unanswered, but these questions do not dominate their narrative, thus indicating their resolved state of mind. For example one mother responded to the question about the causes for the child's difficulties as follows:

> "In the first trimester of the pregnancy I was ill and I took antibiotics. In the past I used to think a lot about this, and I thought that maybe I caused it, but today it's clear to me that it was not something I could control, it just happened."

This mother's preoccupation with the medication she took and the resultant guilt have not disappeared. She does not say that she *knows* the antibiotics were not the cause—but just that it was "something I could not control." The preoccupation and guilt have subsided sufficiently to allow the focus on the present.

Subclassifications of Resolution

As mentioned above, the resolved classification includes three subclassifications, with the first being *resolved–thinking oriented*. Parents in this group acknowledge their feelings around the diagnosis but focus primarily on their thoughts about the process they underwent and express reflections and insight. For example, when describing the day of receiving the diagnosis, one father said (italics emphasize reflective statements):

> "At first we received a diagnosis from the Child Development Center. They told us he has autism. I was very sad, and we decided to get a second opinion—*I think we wanted to hear* that the diagnosis wasn't true. The psychologist we saw was much more optimistic, she wasn't even sure he had PDD. It was a real relief because *that is what I wanted to hear at the time*. Later on it turned out that she was wrong and I was angry with her for misleading us, giving us false hopes. *Today I know* that no one knows exactly the exact diagnosis of these children. I think the whole idea of a "PDD spectrum" is that it is very different from child to child—*but it's hard to understand this at first. You can't grasp it in the beginning*."

This father's resolution is expressed in his capacity to explain the motives underlying the decision to seek a second opinion (wanting to hear the diagnosis was not true), motives that openly refer to the initial shock and difficulty in accepting the harsh diagnosis, but that also put this emotional reaction in a temporal perspective that suggests it has changed. Similarly this father contrasts the initial relief and encouragement following the "optimistic" diagnosis received as a second opinion with the anger he felt when he discovered this optimistic view was unfounded. This father's process orientation and capacity to speak openly about his changing feelings is also evident in his contrasting of his initial difficulties in understanding what it means to "be on the PDD spectrum" and how that has changed with time.

Other resolved parents emphasize the feelings they experienced throughout the process, and are considered *resolved–feeling oriented*. These parents may discuss receiving the diagnosis as a traumatic experience. They may talk about having experienced feelings of depression or doom (e.g., "It was the end of the world for me," "I felt as if I fell into a very deep hole"), and denial or even anger toward those making the diagnosis. However, throughout the interview and especially when asked the "change" question, these parents talk about a meaningful change in their feelings about the diagnosis and describe how they were able to go back to their everyday life. At this point, resolved parents refer to the diagnosis of autism as one part of their lives, but they report they feel their lives are back on course. They support the statements about changes with compelling examples, and their discussion of the positive changes in their feelings is believable, often related to improvements they see in their child's functioning. The following is an example of this subclassification. In response to the question about the day of the diagnosis one mother responded:

> "I was in shock, I felt I was suffocating . . . I sat there and cried, it was very difficult . . . very *very* difficult. That whole day I couldn't stop crying. My husband and I didn't want to talk to anyone. We didn't know how we are going to tell this to our friends and relatives. I think it was the most terrible day of my life. I felt like everything else was unimportant."

But later on, when asked the "change" question the same mother answered:

> "Today I have many moments of pleasure, many hours of pleasure. I see his progress, I see how he develops as a child in general, he is communicating much more, so there is much more room for optimism. Of course things have changed, we see that he is making progress."

The final subclassification involves a focus on what can be done to help the child and is therefore labeled *resolved–action oriented*. These parents may describe receiving the diagnosis as not necessarily very traumatic, but they acknowledge it was difficult. They focus on describing what they have done, are doing, and are planning to do for their child, and also talk briefly about their feelings or thoughts and how they changed. They often describe their initial responses as involving seeking information about the diagnosis that would help them help their child, and finding the right treatment for their child. Thus, while the way they describe their reaction to receiving the diagnosis does not involve focusing on internal thoughts and emotions like the two styles described above, these parents are still considered resolved because they describe a process of change and show acceptance of the diagnosis and of their child. For example, when describing the day of receiving the diagnosis, one mother said:

> "It was not an easy day, I remember coming home and crying. But at the same time—I was finally given a title for the problem of my son, and that in a way was a relief. Now we could start treating and working with him . . . I started to read, to find out about it, to know exactly what it means. My next reaction was just to find him a good place where they can help him and to try and do as much as we could for him."

In conclusion, three main styles of resolution can be identified, reflecting thinking, feeling, or action orientations. In addition, all interviews seen as resolved share three main features: change in feelings over time, acceptance, and suspension of the search for reasons. Significantly, no style is seen as better or as indicating higher levels of, or more robust, resolution. This is important because some clinical approaches may consider certain orientations, such as those focusing on processing of feelings, as indicating "deeper" resolution than those focusing on action. Here all are considered equally resolved because they indicate that parents have revised their internal working model of the child and of the self and are primarily oriented to the present and future. It is also important to mention that there can be overlap between the orientations, and that these are not mutually exclusive categories. For example, an interview can reflect an orientation that is primarily "thinking" but may also include components of "action." In conclusion, the undistorted orientation to the present that characterizes resolved parents is likely to support interactions with their children that are matched to the children's needs. They see and accept the children's difficulties but also the children's unique characteristics that are unrelated to their diagnosis, and therefore are likely to respond appropriately to the children's behaviors.

Unresolved with Respect to the Child's Diagnosis

Unresolved parents have difficulties in revising their internal working models of their child as being a child with a significant developmental disability. The overall impression is that the parent does not accept the child for what he or she is, often portraying a one-sided, unrealistic view of the child. Furthermore, the parent appears to not allow him- or herself to express painful emotions in reaction to the diagnosis or is still absorbed in the initial response to the diagnosis. Both of these positions reflect unbalanced views and feelings toward the child's diagnosis. The unresolved classification is divided into several subclassifications: neutralizing, emotionally overwhelmed, angrily preoccupied, depressed, cognitively distorted, or confused. We describe each next.

The *unresolved–neutralizing* subclassification involves emotional disengagement from the affective meaning of the diagnosis. Such parents can speak about the day on which they received the diagnosis, and some may even recall many details from that day. However, they seem cut off from the full meaning of the emotional experience. They usually do not describe any difficulty or only minimal discomfort after receiving the diagnosis. For example one mother, when asked about her reaction to receiving the diagnosis, said:

> "The truth is that I didn't . . . I heard that some parents, on that day, when they left the doctor's office, received the diagnosis, aahh . . . all their world turned around. I didn't feel like that. I really didn't. I accepted it as it is, I don't know, I didn't cry, no depression, there was nothing, I simply accepted it. . . . We talked to the doctor, he explained to us about it, he was very nice, and we accepted it in a nice way."

The mother refers to receiving the diagnosis in a matter-of-fact manner that seems to minimize the emotional impact of the event. We speculate that such responses represent attempts to gain distance from the painful and anxiety-evoking implications of the diagnosis. Importantly, this mother and others classified as neutralizing show no reflection regarding the defensive nature of this response, or any other indication that they have gained perspective regarding their initial, minimizing reaction. For example, there is no description of a process in which the initial response changed over time. While a neutralizing strategy may help parents cope with the emotions evoked by the diagnosis, it limits their capacity to revise their working model of the child in line with the diagnosis and may therefore lead to parental responses that are mismatched to the child's needs.

Unresolved neutralizing responses bear some similarity to resolved–action-oriented responses; both focus on what parents have done and are doing to help their child. However, neutralizing parents do not refer to their feelings and show no indication of an emotional and cognitive process taking place between receiving the diagnosis and the present. For example one unresolved–neutralizing mother said:

> "First of all I didn't believe he was autistic, I thought they exaggerated. We started looking for the right place for him. . . . Since then, many things changed, we succeeded to enroll him into a special class, which helped him progress a lot."

This mother describes her initial reaction as denial—"I didn't believe he was autistic." This denial is described as the initial response, one that occurred many months prior to the interview, and there is no reference to changes that took place as time passed by. The question of whether this mother still feels her child does not have autism remains unanswered. She moved on to discuss what she did to help her child, but her own reactions and feelings at that time and until the present are absent.

Contrast this to the interview of a father classified as resolved action-oriented who similarly talks about initial denial and the "exaggeration" of the psychologist. He focuses more on actions than on feelings or thoughts, but adopts a process orientation that describes the evolution of his stance from denial to acceptance. He describes the process as follows:

> "At first I was in denial. I thought that the psychologist is exaggerating, but then we got into wanting to help the child. We started reading and looking for the right treatment program for him. Today I am no longer in denial, I talk about it with people, I know he has a problem. I think we found a good treatment program that helps him and he is progressing at his own pace."

While unresolved–neutralizing parents distance themselves from negative affects, other parents, considered *unresolved–emotionally overwhelmed*, are flooded by them. The central characteristic of these parents is that they appear to be overwhelmed by their feelings about the diagnosis of the child, as if still in the midst of mourning the loss of the typically developing child they yearned for. Intense negative feelings such as sadness and anger are expressed, and there is very little or no indication that these feelings have changed over time, or are in the process of changing. In fact, some parents describe their feelings as getting worse, not better. One father said that the day of the diagnosis was difficult, but since then he feels that it has only gotten worse. He describes his family's current circumstances as chaotic, "a loop they are in and can not get out of," and attributes this to having a child with autism. Another mother said:

> "That day was a horrible shock. To tell you the truth I didn't think about autism at all. I felt as if my world has been destroyed, I simply saw black everywhere. I didn't understand why this happened to me. People think I'm strong but I don't feel that way. Every day is a struggle, just seeing mothers walking with their children makes me sad. Today more and more and more, it just keeps intensifying—I pity my child."

Both parents portray a difficult, harsh reality regarding their child and family. It seems as if having a child with autism colors every moment of the day and every aspect of their emotional experience, and this pervasive feeling leaves little room for more positive experiences. The child is seen primarily, if not solely, through the lens of the diagnosis with no mentioning of positive or rewarding aspects. While here the parents do not seem to have difficulties incorporating the child's diagnosis into their view of him or her, they have great difficulties forming a balanced, individualized view of the child that gives a place to aspects other than the child's pathology. This is likely to limit their capacity to correctly read the child's signals and appropriately respond to the child's needs.

The flooding of feelings may also be manifested in the length of the interview responses. Such interviews are overelaborated, excessively detailed, or include repetitions. Some parents show associative thinking and have difficulty staying on the topic, to the point that the interviewer has to help the parent and refocus him or her in order to complete the response.

Some emotionally overwhelmed parents blame themselves for the child's situation. When asked about the possible reasons for their child's condition one mother described a direct relationship between postponing a certain medical test and her child's autism:

> "The doctor sent us to do this test, but the same week I had a business trip and we decided to postpone the test for a week. Until this day I am angry at myself for doing that, who knows—maybe things would have been different with him."

Another mother blamed herself repeatedly and said:

> "I feel it is because of me. When he was little I didn't invest myself in raising him, those years were a difficult period in our family, and I also felt that everybody around me was blaming me—maybe they were right."

Both mothers feel a heavy load of responsibility and guilt regarding their child's condition. The question about parental feelings of responsibility is particularly complex in the case of autism because research regarding the etiology of autism has not provided definite answers to date. This leaves room for a wide range of attempts by parents to figure out the possible causes for their child's condition. These two examples suggest difficulties in resolution due to the self-blame, certainty, and rigidity associated with the explanations suggested, not the explanations per se. Both mothers are sure that specific actions on their part led to the child's autism, and these thoughts arise repeatedly during the interview. While these mothers are heavily invested in their children, their guilt may so preoccupy their minds that it is likely to interfere with their capacity to free up the mental and emotional resources needed in order to be emotionally available to their children.

An additional manifestation of the emotionally overwhelmed subclassification involves speaking about the day of the diagnosis as if it was very recent, or even using the present tense when describing that day. It is important to note that all the interviews described in this chapter were conducted at least 1 year after the diagnosis was made, and often even much longer than that. These parents seem to relive the day of the diagnosis with all its intensity and immediacy in the present. For example, one mother said, "I remember this day as if it was yesterday," and then went on to describe the room in which she received the diagnosis, specifying where each person sat and citing the words of the formal letter given to her. The stress or trauma of the day are relived in the present, and each day lived from that moment on appears to be shadowed by the diagnosis.

An additional unresolved subclassification is labeled *unresolved–angry preoccupation*. These parents express anger toward the interviewer or, more often, toward professionals who gave them the diagnosis or are treating their child, possibly to divert attention from the reality of the diagnosis. One mother who did not agree with the diagnosis and was angry for the way the family was treated by the diagnostic team talked about the day of the diagnosis and said:

"They only said, 'Not good. Not good.' It was terrible. I couldn't stop crying. . . . I didn't want to return to that place. How can I believe in their treatment? I could have had an accident on the way home because of them. Do you know how much I cried? I am telling you—do you know how I left that place? I couldn't walk! Do you know that till this day they never called us to see how he is doing! Even the psychologist who is treating him now was angry at them and couldn't understand how they did such a thing to me."

This same mother, when asked the "change" question started to describe her child's progress, but immediately returned to talk about her anger:

"I can see how much he progressed. If you saw him today you wouldn't believe it—so to ruin everything for me? And to tell me . . . ? Why? You know what, when I think about it, I don't even want to talk about it."

It is apparent that this mother is still intensely angry. This mother's anger is fueled in part by her fierce protectiveness of her child. However, because the anger is so intense and pervasive it does not enhance her availability to her child but rather shifts her attention away. As with the unresolved–overwhelmed pattern described above, the concern is that the anger so preoccupies the mother that it reduces her availability to the child. This is not to say that some resolved parents do not express anger. For example, a resolved parent may express anger at a professional who they feel did not behave appropriately, but this anger will be more modulated and focused on the past, and will not color the view of the child.

Other parents who are unresolved are classified as *unresolved-depressed*. This may be seen in their passivity and sadness during the interview, and in the content of their answers—they speak about being depressed and helpless, and report on a great deal of crying. For example:

"After receiving the diagnosis I was depressed for a long time. . . . I had symptoms of depression. I shouldn't say this, but my life will never be the same. I don't think I will ever be a happy person again. . . . Even if I'll have a new house, a new car, I have a wonderful husband and another wonderful child, but let's face it, I will never be happy deep inside."

In this example receiving the diagnosis leaves the mother empty, hopeless, and with a feeling of eternal sadness. Here again the diagnosis is the central focus, leaving the mother with no energy to see other, more positive aspects of her child. Another characteristic of these parents is their tendency to blame themselves and answer the "causes" question with reference to self-blame.

The final two subclassifications, *cognitive distortions* and *disorganized–confused*, are less common. The first refers to parents who distort the events or information about the diagnosis and their child. They may deny the diagnosis or have unrealistic expectations as to the future of their child ("I'm sure my child will study in a regular class and grow up to be anything he wants, even a pilot"). For example when asked about the first time he noticed his child's difficulty, one father said:

> "There was one kindergarten teacher that said that there is something wrong with him, but I absolutely did not agree with her. I insisted that he was OK until I had no choice because no kindergarten would accept him."

The father refused to go to the diagnostic meetings and said, in response to the "change" question:

> "I still believe that it is only temporary. I can't ignore that there is a problem if society sees it that way, you can not escape society, but I do not accept that there is a problem, and anyway I still insist that he will attend a regular class."

The other subclassification, *disorganized–confused,* refers to parents whose incoherent or associative speech makes it difficult for the listener to understand the meaning of their answers. For example, one father said:

> "I'm telling you the truth, even when the child was young when I went to work he also, he—he has a very strong affection to me and then he had epilepsy, the epilepsy seizure doesn't matter you put these things the simple way, I don't know these things . . . "

In sum, the unresolved subclassifications are all thought to reflect the difficulties parents have with coming to terms with their children's diagnoses and revising their working models of their children in light of these diagnoses. As in the subclassifications of the resolved group, here too all of the subclassifications are considered equally unresolved—reflecting different parental styles in dealing with this immense challenge.

THE REACTION TO DIAGNOSIS INTERVIEW: RESEARCH EVIDENCE

In this section we summarize our research findings from our preschool study of mothers of young boys with an autism spectrum disorder (ASD) and from our family study of mothers and fathers of children with an ASD. In both studies, we employed the RDI. We begin our summary with descriptive results regarding the percentage of parents classified resolved or unresolved.

Our findings showed that 33% of mothers of children with an ASD were classified as resolved in our preschool study, and 37% of mothers and 52% of fathers were classified as resolved in our family study. The rates pertaining to mothers are somewhat lower than those reported by Pianta and colleagues (1996), who reported that 56% of the mothers of children with epilepsy and 46% of the mothers of children with cerebral palsy were classified as resolved. Comparing the studies suggests that resolution is perhaps more easily achieved by mothers of children diagnosed with the relatively mild diagnosis of epilepsy than by mothers of children diagnosed with the more severe diagnosis of autism/PDD.

If rates of resolution are higher when less severe diagnoses are concerned, is it also the case that resolution will be more likely for less severe cases *within* the spectrum of ASD? To address this question we examined whether the resolved or unresolved status of the parent is associated with the severity of the child's condition. We examined this question by exploring the associations between children's IQs and level of functioning (which combines cognitive functioning and attainment of age-expected daily living skills) and the RDI classifications of their parents. We also examined the link between severity of the diagnosis (a PDD NOS diagnosis representing a milder form of the disorder compared to autistic disorder) and resolution. No significant associations were found in either comparison, suggesting that RDI classifications are not associated with the severity of the child's condition. Similar findings were obtained by Pianta and colleagues (1996), who reported that severity of the child's diagnosis was not associated with parental resolution status in families of children with cerebral palsy or epilepsy.

Thus, RDI classifications are not related to the severity of the child's diagnosis but rather appear to be reflections of how parents cope with the diagnosis. As demonstrated by some of the examples above, it is possible to speak in a resolved manner regarding a child whose functioning is relatively low, for example, by highlighting the strengths of the child or the gains made in treatment. Along these lines, a relatively high level of functioning of the child does not insure acceptance or resolution. For example, one mother of a particularly high-functioning child with autism found the discrepancy between the high cognitive functioning and the poor communication skills particularly confusing and hard to accept, resulting in an interview classified as unresolved.

Our next question was whether resolution is a function of the time that has passed since the diagnosis was made. Does time "heal the wounds" so that parents are more likely to be resolved if a longer time has elapsed since they received the diagnosis? Pianta and colleagues (1996) reported no associations between the time elapsed since the diagnosis and resolution, and the same findings were obtained in our studies. The family study was particularly important for examining this issue because many of the children were older than those in the preschool study, with a longer time passing since the diagnosis was given. The findings indicate that the passage of time in and of itself does not ensure resolution.

This is an important finding and one that raises concern. Combined with the relatively high proportion of unresolved parents it suggests that difficulties in resolving the diagnosis are both relatively common and relatively stable. Simply put: many parents have difficulties coming to terms with the diagnosis of their child, and these difficulties do not seem to "go away" as time goes by. These findings point to the need for interventions designed to promote resolution, and this issue will be discussed further later.

Up to this point we have focused on correlates of the RDI classifications, and we move now to results pertaining to what is perhaps the central issue: the implications of parental resolution for the child and the parent–child relationship. As mentioned earlier, prior work on resolution (e.g., Main & Hesse, 1990) was motivated primarily by seeking to understand the negative implications that lack of resolution may bear on parental behavior toward the child. The findings of Pianta and colleagues (1996) supported this notion by revealing associations between lack of resolution and insecure attachment in children with epilepsy and children with cerebral palsy. The results of our preschool study also support this notion, by linking resolution of the diagnosis to mothers' sensitive caregiving behavior.

Specifically, we focused on mothers' sensitivity (Biringen & Robinson, 1991) as rated from observations in three different interactional contexts: free play, structured play, and social play. According to Biringen, Robinson, and Emde (1993), sensitivity involves accurate reading of children's emotional signals and prompt, flexible, and appropriate responses, all within the context of a positive emotional climate. Because resolution involves acceptance of the diagnosis while also seeing the child *beyond* the diagnosis we expected that mothers classified as resolved would be rated as more sensitive than those classified as unresolved. Our results confirmed this expectation. In fact, not only were the mothers classified as resolved sensitive *relative* to those classified unresolved, their mean sensitivity score fell within the range considered by the scale developers as "sensitive." This finding is very important given the immense challenges that children with autism have in reciprocal social interaction, challenges that make sensitive maternal responses all the more difficult. Significantly, the association between resolution and sensitivity held even when children's level of functioning was statistically controlled. Similar results were also found with ratings of maternal structuring, indicating that mothers classified as resolved structured the interaction with their child more optimally than those classified as unresolved, again, regardless of the child's level of functioning.

These results link maternal resolution to maternal behavior with the child; we next asked if resolution is also associated with *children's* behavior during interactions with their mothers. We hypothesized that children of resolved mothers will be more responsive to their mothers and more involving of their mothers during interactions compared to children whose mothers are unresolved. The reasoning behind this hypothesis was that children's responsiveness and involvement are optimal when they experience the parent's behavior as congruent with their needs and matched to their signals, as is expected from the parenting behavior of resolved parents. Also, it was particularly important to examine children's responsiveness and involvement because these represent areas of vulnerability for children with autism (Biringen, Fidler, Barrett, & Kubicek, 2005).

Children's behavior was coded from the same interactions described above. The findings revealed that mothers classified as resolved had children who were more responsive to them and who were more involving of them during interaction compared to children of mothers classified as unresolved. These results applied only to children classified as "low functioning," however. As mentioned above, this designation reflects children's overall low cognitive and functional skills, and applied to the majority of children in the study (73%). Perhaps the more vulnerable, low-functioning children are particularly sensitive to lack of resolution of the parent, resulting in lower involvement of the parent and responsiveness to the parent.

How can we understand the links between resolution and maternal as well as child behavior? The essence of lack of resolution involves failures or difficulties in revising the parent's working model of the child in light of the child's diagnosis and the limitations that it implies. The parent fails to "realign the model with the new reality," to use Bowlby's phrase. This mismatch between the working model of the child in the mind of the parent and the child in reality may interfere with the capacity of the parent to read the child's signals correctly and respond in appropriate ways. For example, the parent may respond more to the "wished-for" child than the actual child by attributing to the child capabilities that are far beyond his or her actual abilities. As a result these parents may experience more difficulties in meeting the child at the level on which the child is functioning, and from the point of view of the child this can be experienced as frustrating or confusing, lowering his or her responsiveness and involvement. Alternatively, parents may defensively see the child only through the perspective of the diagnosis and have difficulties seeing the child as a whole person. This may lead to dismissal of the child's more "normal" emotional and developmental needs such as the need to feel secure, to play, or to enjoy unstructured time.

While these explanations focus on the impact of the parent on the child, effects of the child on the parent are also possible. For example, perhaps it is more difficult to be resolved with respect to the child's diagnosis when the child is particularly unresponsive and not involving? Intervention studies can be particularly useful to clarify this issue. For example, a study that targets parents who are unresolved and demonstrates that interventions designed to foster resolution in the parent lead to positive shifts in maternal and child behavior during interaction may be helpful. We discuss the issue of intervention next.

RESOLUTION OF THE DIAGNOSIS
AND INTERVENTION

Intervention with parents who are unresolved with respect to the child's diagnosis first requires identifying this state of mind in parents. Can resolution be assessed in the "real world," when the administration the RDI is not possible or practical? One answer is that administering the RDI in clinical settings is not necessarily impossible. The RDI is not too long or time consuming, and typically requires about 15 minutes to administer. The general nature of the questions presented in the RDI is not very different from questions parents are asked at intake, when they first bring their children to a clinic or agency. The RDI can therefore be part of a broader interview or assessment.

Using the RDI questions is not only possible but can have added value beyond routine questioning. For example, many clinicians might ask parents when they first noticed that their child had difficulties (the first RDI question) as part of routine history taking. However, they may not necessarily ask other RDI questions, such as those about the feelings during the time of diagnosis, the change in these feelings, or parents' thoughts about the reasons for the child's condition. These questions are crucial in order to learn not only about the parent's emotional reaction but also about the process the parent has gone through since the time of the diagnosis—a crucial aspect of resolution.

The RDI can also be used in clinical practice to encourage parents to speak directly about the child's diagnosis and express their feelings about the topic. The questions carry the message that feelings and thoughts regarding the child's diagnosis are not just something the parent needs to deal with on his or her own, in order to "clear the way" for intervention with the child. Rather, discussing these feelings is part and parcel of the intervention with the child and the parents, and a legitimate and important topic for discussion and mutual work. The wording of the questions is carefully designed to be direct, yet open and neutral. For example, the questions do not suggest that changes in feelings regarding the diagnosis over time *have* to occur, only that they might. Also, questions are not phrased to ask about guilt, but rather to open up a discussion regarding possible reasons for the child's diagnosis.

Legitimizing discussion of the parent's feelings is important, because many times the urgent needs of the child capture the entire "space" of intervention efforts. Inadvertently parents and professionals may collude in not talking about the parent's feelings and focus only on trying to help the child. This is fueled by the child's multiple urgent needs, and by the fact that bringing up potentially painful memories, thoughts, and emotions can be difficult for both the parents and the therapist and may therefore be avoided.

We discussed the feasibility and usefulness of *administering* the RDI in clinical contexts, but the question of *coding* the RDI in such contexts–that is, of concluding whether the parent is resolved or unresolved—is more complex. Our experience with the RDI suggests that correct use requires specific training. Such training involves in-depth familiarity with the coding manual, hands-on experience in coding interviews while receiving feedback, and addressing the many inherent complexities of interviews that do not fall neatly into the classifications. Overall clinical impressions based on cursory familiarity with the coding system cannot replace such training. Yet, familiarity with the coding system, such as through the examples provided in this chapter, can help clinicians fine-tune their understanding of the parents and of where parents are with respect to the resolution process. This enhanced understanding is probably more important clinically than classifying a parent as resolved or unresolved (Slade, 2004).

Our second question about intervention focuses on the best "port of entry" for intervention. Should interventions be "top-down," focusing on parents' difficulties revising their internal working models and working through their defensive strategies? Such interventions are based on the premise that helping parents come to terms with the diagnosis of their child will facilitate their caregiving to the child. Alternatively, interventions can operate in a "bottom-up" direction, facilitating sensitive interactions between the child and the parent, which in turn can help parents more easily achieve a resolved state of mind.

Answers to these questions require further research that is not yet available, but we can point to some possible directions. Stern's writing about "ports of entry" (Stern, 1995) emphasizes how "entrance" through different ports, that is, intervening at different levels, such as at the representational system (in our case, resolution) or at the behavioral system (in our case, parental behavior), may yield similar therapeutic outcomes. Stern explains that this is because the systems are interlinked and changes in one system lead to changes in the other. This suggests that it may not matter which port of entry is chosen. However, even if this is the case, it may still be that entrance from one port is more efficient than from another, depending on the parent's style of coping with emotional issues.

For example, most of the unresolved mothers in our preschool study were of the emotionally overwhelmed subtype. Remembering the time of the diagnosis and thinking about their child overwhelmed these mothers with grief, sadness, and pain. It seems that these mothers had no difficulties opening up and talking about these painful issues but had difficulties containing the negative affects and achieving a sense of regulation and coherence. With such parents, it may be that intervention that focuses on the grief process in relation to the diagnosis may be beneficial. Other unresolved mothers in our study showed a neutralizing style. Attempting to approach their internal experience regarding the child's diagnosis is likely to engender resistance because it does not seem to be consistent with their style. However, focusing on the interaction with the child and emphasizing understanding the child's special needs may be more effective. As is always the case in clinical work, sensitivity to the parent and trying to best understand each parent's perspective are always of prime importance. Resolution, like mourning, may take many different shapes and progress through various pathways, requiring that interventions consider this variability.

Parents of children with special needs work with many professionals who assist them with their child's disability, only a few of whom focus on their psychological responses. These may include occupational and speech therapists, pediatricians, special educators, and so on. We believe that raising the awareness for *all* professionals working with children with special needs to the resolution process may be helpful for several reasons. First, such awareness can help normalize reactions that may be difficult to understand. For example, understanding that strong expressions of pain, guilt or anger, or avoidance of issues related to the child's diagnosis are expected grief reactions can enhance their acceptance. Sympathetic listening to such expressions can facilitate resolution.

Awareness can also facilitate empathy with the parents' experience. For example, behaviors that are labeled as "denial" or lack of cooperation can be reframed as reflecting outward expressions of an underlying, painful resolution process. This reframing can help professionals adopt accepting, emotionally containing responses. Such responses are not only likely to facilitate resolution but also likely to improve the relationships between professionals and parents. Sometimes they may even enhance the effectiveness of the intervention work, particularly in interventions in which therapists work with the parent and child.

In sum, the resolution process of parents of children who receive significant developmental diagnoses is of profound importance both for the parents and for the children. Resolution enhances parents' capacity to help children maximize their developmental potential within the limits imposed by their disabilities. In a parallel fashion, professionals working with these parents are uniquely positioned to play a very important facilitative role supporting parents in the often difficult and painful resolution process.

ACKNOWLEDGMENT

This research was supported by the Israel Science Foundation (Grant Nos. 824/2002 and 540/3).

REFERENCES

Biringen, Z., Fidler, D. J., Barrett, K. C., & Kubicek, L. (2005). Applying the emotional availability scales to children with disabilities. *Infant Mental Health Journal, 26*(4), 369–391.

Biringen, Z., & Robinson, J. (1991). Emotional availability in mother–child interactions: A reconceptualization for research. *American Journal of Orthopsychiatry, 61,* 258–271.

Biringen, Z., Robinson, J., & Emde B. (1993). *The Emotional Availability Scales.* Unpublished manuscript, University of Colorado Health Sciences Center, Denver.

Bowlby, J. (1980). *Attachment and loss: Vol. 3. Loss.* New York: Basic Books.

Dolev, S. (2005). *Maternal insightfulness and resolution of the diagnosis among mothers of young boys with ASD.* Unpublished doctoral dissertation, University of Haifa, Israel.

Lyons-Ruth, K., & Spielman, E. (2004). Disorganized infant attachment strategies and helpless-fearful profiles of parenting: Integrating attachment research with clinical intervention. *Infant Mental Health Journal, 25,* 318–335.

Main, M., & Hesse, E. (1990). Parents' unresolved traumatic experiences are related to infant disorganized attachment status: Is frightened and/or frightening parental behavior the linking mechanism? In M. Greenberg, D. Cicchetti, & E. M. Cummings (Eds.), *Attachment in the preschool years: Theory, research and intervention* (pp. 161–184). Chicago: University of Chicago Press.

Main, M., Kaplan, N., & Cassidy, J. (1985). Security in infancy, childhood and adulthood: A move to the level of representation. In I. Bretherton & E. Waters (Eds.), Growing points of attachment theory and research. *Monographs of the Society for Research in Child Development, 50*(1–2, Serial No. 209), 66–104.

Marvin, R. S., & Pianta, R. C. (1996). Mothers' reactions to their child's diagnosis: Relations with security of attachment. *Journal of Clinical Child Psychology*, *25*, 436–445.

Pianta, R. C., & Marvin R. S. (1992). *The reaction to diagnosis interview.* Unpublished material, University of Virginia, Charlottesville.

Pianta, R. C., & Marvin R. S. (1993). *Manual for classification of the reaction to diagnosis interview.* Unpublished material, University of Virginia, Charlottesville.

Pianta, R. C., Marvin, R. S., Britner, P. A., & Borowitz, K. C. (1996). Mothers' resolution of their children's diagnosis: Organized patterns of caregiving representations. *Journal of Infant Mental Health*, *17*, 239–256.

Pianta, R. C., Marvin, R. S., & Morog, M. C. (1999). Resolving the past and present: Relations with attachment organization. In J. Solomon & C. C. George (Eds.), *Attachment disorganization* (pp. 379–398). New York: Guilford Press.

Salomon, S., Yirmiya, N., Oppenheim, D., Koren-Karie, N., Shulman, C., & Levi, S. (2006, June). *Resolution regarding the child's diagnosis among parents of children with autism spectrum disorders.* Poster presented at the International Meeting for Autism Research, Montreal, Canada.

Slade, A. (2004). Move from categories to process: Attachment phenomena and clinical evaluation. *Infant Mental Health Journal*, *25*, 269–283.

Stern, D. (1995). *The motherhood constellation.* New York: Basic Books.

van IJzendoorn, M. H., Schuengel, C., & Bakermans-Kranenburg, M. K. (1999). Disorganized attachment in early childhood: Meta-analysis of precursors, concomitants and sequelae. *Development and Psychopathology*, *11*, 225–249.

PART II

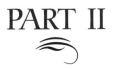

Attachment Theory and Psychotherapy

CHAPTER SIX

Attachment and Trauma

An Integrated Approach to Treating
Young Children Exposed to Family Violence

AMY L. BUSCH and ALICIA F. LIEBERMAN

Young children instinctively rely on their caregivers for protection from danger (Bowlby, 1969/1982). When children experience a traumatic event during their early years, their trust in their attachment figures' ability to protect them is drastically challenged. Traumatic experiences shatter the "protective shield" (Freud, 1920/1955) that parents normatively provide for their children, threatening the core of the attachment relationship. Frightening events also can dysregulate the parent–child relationship by triggering posttraumatic stress reactions in both the child and the adult, hindering the child's ability to seek comfort from the parent and the parent's reciprocal ability to provide reassurance. The deleterious impact of traumatic events on attachment extends beyond infancy into the preschool years.

At the same time, children's ability to recover from traumatic experiences is influenced by the quality of their attachments. A child with secure attachment relationships is likely to trust that others will be available in times of need and that he or she is worthy of their help, and these attitudes may facilitate the child's readiness and ability to seek assistance. Conversely, a child with insecure attachments may be more vulnerable to trauma because the child lacks the inner resources and the emotional support needed to cope with overwhelming circumstances (Belsky & Fearon, 2002; Toth & Cicchetti, 1996). A "dual lens" that integrates both attachment and trauma theory is necessary in clinical situations to help restore the developmental momentum of traumatized young children (Lieberman & Amaya-Jackson, 2005; Lieberman & Van Horn, 2005).

The following example illustrates a child's emotional stance toward her father after she witnessed his violence toward her mother:

> Maria, age 5, was drawing a picture of her family. The clinician asked Maria to tell her about the drawing, and Maria answered, "This is me, this is my mommy, and this is my brother." The clinician said, "I see. But what about your father—he's not in the picture?" The little girl replied, "Sometimes I forget about my daddy because he was mean to my mommy."

Why might this little girl want to "forget" about her father? Maria and her younger brother, Anthony, age 3, had witnessed several incidents of domestic violence between their parents. In omitting her father from her family drawing, Maria may have been showing her desire to avoid the memories of her father's frightening behavior, just as she wanted to avoid him while the violence was taking place. Avoidance has been identified both as an indicator of insecure attachment (Ainsworth, Blehar, Waters, & Wall, 1978) and as a symptom of posttraumatic stress disorder (PTSD) in adults as well as in young children (American Psychiatric Association, 1994; Zero to Three, 2005).

In this chapter, we recommend that clinicians use a combined attachment and trauma framework when intervening with children who have experienced domestic violence and other traumatic life events. We begin by identifying domestic violence as a traumatic stressor that affects children's attachment relationships with their caregivers, both directly and through potential posttraumatic stress responses in children and caregivers. We then discuss how the quality of children's attachment relationships can moderate the impact of trauma on their mental health. In the second half of the chapter, we present the case of Maria, Anthony, and their mother to highlight how clinicians might use an integrated attachment and trauma framework in assessing and intervening with traumatized young children and their caregivers.

DOMESTIC VIOLENCE: TRAUMA WITHIN
THE ATTACHMENT–CAREGIVING SYSTEM

Domestic violence is a prime example of a situation in which attachment and trauma are inextricably linked for a child. The basic premise of attachment theory is that children have a biological predisposition to seek out their caregivers for protection from danger (Bowlby, 1969/ 1982). Their caregivers' pattern of responsiveness teaches children the degree to which they can consistently rely on their caregivers to relieve their fears and ensure their safety. Children whose caregivers generally are responsive to their distress tend to develop secure attachment relationships, while children whose caregivers are neglectful, rejecting, or inconsistently responsive to their vulnerability tend to develop insecure attachment relationships with them (Ainsworth et al., 1978).

In some circumstances, caregivers may be more than neglectful or unresponsive, they actually may appear frightening to a young child. Young children who fear their caregivers are faced with "fright without solution"—the paradox that their potential source of protection is also their source of fear (Hesse & Main, 2000). As a result, children's attachment relationships with these caregivers may become disorganized. In the Strange Situation procedure (Ainsworth et al., 1978), disorganized infants display contradictory approach and avoidance behaviors, appear unnaturally still or frozen, or show other signs of disorientation when interacting with their caregivers. By age 6, disorganized attachment appears to take the form of controlling behavior with caregivers. Some controlling children are punitive, commanding their parents to do things, while others seem excessively caregiving of their parents (Main & Cassidy, 1988). Their caregivers, in turn, often appear helpless within the parent–child relationship (e.g., Lyons-Ruth, Bronfman, & Atwood, 1999).

Domestic violence is a strong risk factor for disorganized attachment in early childhood (Zeanah et al., 1999). An attachment perspective suggests several reasons for this association. First, witnessing domestic violence between caregivers shatters the child's trust that the parent will not cause pain and injury and will protect the child from danger. Seeing one's caregiver harmed or injured may be overwhelmingly terrifying for a young child, and that fear may become linked with the child's mental representation of either the perpetrator or the victim of the violence (Lieberman, 2004; Lieberman & Amaya-Jackson, 2005). This fear of the caregiver may then disorganize the attachment relationship with that person.

There also may be indirect pathways to disorganized attachment among children who have witnessed domestic violence. For example, mothers' lack of resolution regarding past trauma on the Adult Attachment Interview (AAI; George, Kaplan, & Main, 1996) has being linked to disorganized attachment in their infants (van IJzendoorn, Schuengel, & Bakermans-Kranenburg, 1999). In our own sample of battered mothers, 53% were classified on the AAI as having unresolved loss or abuse (Busch & Lieberman, 2006). Mothers who remain unresolved regarding their own past traumatic experiences tend to appear frightened or frightening when interacting with their young children (Schuengel, Bakermans-Kranenburg, & van IJzendoorn, 1999). For example, some unresolved mothers loom aggressively at their infants while playing, while others freeze or seem to enter dissociative-like states during parent–child interactions (Hesse & Main, 2000). These frightening parental behaviors are associated with disorganized attachment in children.

There is also evidence that battered women are at higher risk of abusing their own children (Osofsky, 2003), and maltreatment has been directly linked to disorganized attachment (van IJzendoorn et al., 1999). Of course, these two parenting paths toward disorganized attachment are not mutually exclusive: given the intergenerational transmission of childhood abuse, it is likely that mothers who maltreat their infants were themselves abused as children and remain unresolved regarding those experiences. Thus, in addition to directly abusing their children, these mothers may display the more subtle, frightening behaviors associated with unresolved loss or abuse.

The Contribution of a Trauma Lens: Posttraumatic Stress Responses in Child and Caregiver

By using a trauma lens, clinicians may identify an additional pathway to disorganized child–parent relationships, beyond those identified in the attachment literature. Witnessing domestic violence may constitute a traumatic stressor for a child, defined as "direct experience, witnessing, or confrontation with an event or events that involve actual or threatened death or serious injury to the child or others, or a threat to the psychological or physical integrity of the child or others" (Zero to Three, 2005, p. 19). As a result of this traumatic experience, children may develop PTSD. A diagnosis of PTSD is appropriate when, following trauma, children display symptoms that are sufficiently intense and pervasive to interfere with their development and that persist for at least 1 month (Zero to Three, 2005). There are three main diagnostic criteria for PTSD in children:

1. *Reexperiencing the traumatic event,* as evidenced by posttraumatic play, repeated nightmares, distress at exposure to reminders of the event.
2. *Numbing of responsiveness or interference with developmental momentum,* manifested by restricted range of affect, diminished interest in play, efforts to avoid activities, places, or people linked to the trauma.
3. *Increased arousal,* including sleep difficulties, attention problems, hypervigilance, exaggerated startle response, increased irritability or temper tantrums.

In addition to these three symptom clusters, other behaviors are considered associated features of PTSD in children, such as the loss of previously acquired developmental skills, aggression toward others, new fears such as separation anxiety, and age-inappropriate sexual behaviors.

PTSD rates are as high as 40% among child witnesses of domestic violence (Chemtob & Carlson, 2004), and children appear to have more severe PTSD symptoms in response to witnessing domestic violence than to frightening events not involving threats to their attachment figures (Scheeringa & Zeanah, 1995). However, parents are often unaware of the effects that trauma can have on a young child, because of guilt over their own involvement in the traumatic event, their mistaken belief that young children are too immature to notice or understand the experience, or their own posttraumatic stress reactions (Lieberman & Van Horn, 2005; Pynoos, Steinberg, & Piacentini, 1999). As a result, parents may misinterpret children's trauma symptoms as oppositional behavior, attention-deficit/hyperactivity disorder, or lack of love on the children's part. This can lead to mutual alienation, miscommunication, a failure to protect, and eventual disorganization of the attachment system (Lieberman, 2004; Lieberman & Amaya-Jackson, 2005; Lyons-Ruth & Jacobvitz, 1999). This may partly explain why some infants appear securely attached to their caregivers but also display momentarily disorganized behavior with them. At least some of these infants may have had a history of responsive caregiving that became disrupted when a traumatic experience, such as domestic violence, injected new fear into the child–parent relationship.

Using a Dual Lens in Conceptualizing Children's Symptoms Following Trauma

Clinicians may note that some of the markers and correlates of disorganized/ controlling attachment behavior in infancy and preschool years are similar to the features of PTSD in children, such as frozen postures, dissociation, aggression, affect dysregulation, cognitive delays, and physiological alterations (for reviews of this research, see Lyons-Ruth & Jacobvitz, 1999; van IJzendoorn et al., 1999). Although to our knowledge, there has been no systematic empirical investigation of this issue to date, theoretical and clinical work suggests that these two constructs may be related (Lieberman, 2004; Lieberman & Amaya-Jackson, 2005). Problems with exploration and learning are associated with both disorganized attachment relationships and posttraumatic stress responses in children. If a caregiver is frightening (i.e., the domestic violence perpetrator) or frightened and helpless (i.e., the victim), then the child may experience fewer of the supportive interactions that normally facilitate learning. In addition, children who must accommodate to the emotional demands of relating to a frightening or helpless parent may deploy their cognitive and emotional resources away from exploration of the environment and learning and toward monitoring of the parent's behavior (Moss, St-Laurent, & Parent, 1999). From a trauma perspective, children's developmental progress can be interrupted when they experience extreme fear during the same period that new developmental milestones are being achieved (Pynoos et al., 1999). Children exposed to high levels of domestic violence tend to score significantly lower on intelligence tests than nonexposed children (Koenen, Moffitt, Caspi, Taylor, & Purcell, 2003). PTSD symptoms, particularly high levels of arousal, may be the mechanism that explains some of these cognitive effects (Stamper & Lieberman, 2006).

The Quality of Attachment Influences Children's Response to Trauma

Although domestic violence and other traumatic events can affect the quality of attachment, the attachment system also can influence a child's response to trauma. Lyons-Ruth and colleagues (Lyons-Ruth et al., 1999) have proposed a "relationship-diathesis" model in which recovery from trauma depends on both the nature of the trauma, such as its suddenness, intensity, developmental timing, and involvement of attachment figures, and the quality of the child's attachment relationships. Consistent with this model, support from caregivers appears to mitigate the negative impact of trauma on children and improve their ability to resolve PTSD symptoms (Cohen, Mannarino, Berliner, & Deblinger, 2000; Cook et al., 2005). Secure attachment relationships also appear protective in the face of cumulative stressors including maternal depression, marital problems, and poverty (Belsky & Fearon, 2000), and are linked to better regulation of physiological stress responses (see Schuder & Lyons-Ruth, 2004, for a review). These findings highlight the important role that the caregiving relationship plays in young children's ability to manage both psychological and physiological responses to trauma, and they suggest that by enhancing the quality of the attachment relationship, clinicians might improve children's ability to cope with traumatic life events. In the following section, we discuss the use of a relationship-focused intervention model to help children recover from traumatic experiences.

USING THE ATTACHMENT RELATIONSHIP TO FACILITATE CHILDREN'S RECOVERY FROM TRAUMA

The interplay of attachment and trauma suggests that intervention for infants, toddlers, and preschoolers who have experienced domestic violence and other traumatic events logically follows a child–parent model. Child–parent psychotherapy (CPP) is founded on the basic premises of attachment and psychodynamic theories, which posit that the parent–child relationship is central to shaping personality development in the early years, and that effective intervention for young children's social-emotional difficulties should focus on this attachment–caregiving system (Lieberman & Van Horn, 2005). When working with families who have experienced family violence or another trauma, the child–parent psychotherapist approaches that trauma as an experience that has profound effects on the child, the mother, and their relationship. While CPP may be conducted with any primary caregiver (mother, father, grandparent, adoptive parent, etc.), we will refer to the caregiver as the mother for purposes of this chapter.

Assessing Trauma and Attachment–Caregiving Relationships in the Family

The first step in CPP involves assessing the child, the mother, and the quality of their relationship. Prior to beginning treatment, the clinician meets the mother alone to learn about her child's history of trauma and psychological symptoms. Knowing as many details as possible about the trauma guides the clinician in choosing appropriate toys for the treatment, and it helps the clinician make connections between the child's play and his or her actual experience during the therapy.

We also recommend that the clinician assess the mother's history of trauma and her symptoms because the mother is a crucial member of the treatment and mothers' mental health directly impacts their ability to care for their children (e.g., Lieberman, Van Horn, & Ozer, 2005). In addition, because parents' ways of thinking about their own childhood experiences influences their parenting of their children (see Hesse, 1999, for a review of this research), we recommend assessing the mother's attachment history. Although we have used the AAI (George, Kaplan, & Main, 1996) in our treatment outcome research, clinicians also may use clinical interviews to assess mothers' childhood experiences and to identify defensive patterns, such as idealization, projection, and isolation of affect, that may characterize parents' psychological functioning and influence their perceptions of their children.

The therapeutic focus of CPP is the relationship between the child and caregiver. The clinician listens closely to the way that the mother describes her relationship with her child during the assessment phase, looking for helpful ports of entry for intervention during treatment. In the final part of the assessment, mother and child are observed playing together using toys, games, and puzzles provided by the clinician. They then participate in a separation and reunion task that is based on the Strange Situation but adapted to the child's age (Ainsworth et al., 1978; Crowell, Feldman, & Ginsberg, 1988). This part of the assessment provides information on a number of domains of the parent–child relationship, such as their capacity to find pleasure in each other, the child's compliance with parental direction, the parent's ability to follow the child's lead in play, how the parent and child manage the potentially stressful experience of separation in an unfamiliar environment (the clinic playroom), and how the child uses the parent for security upon return.

Attachment and Trauma-Focused Goals of Child–Parent Psychotherapy

The primary goal of CPP with traumatized children is to promote and restore developmental progress by helping the child and the parent create a joint narrative of the traumatic event, to place the trauma in the larger context of living, and to find ways of relating and communicating that promote safety, trust, and enjoyment of age-appropriate pursuits (Lieberman & Van Horn, 2005, p. 7). Interventions may take various forms, but they generally have the following aims: (1) increasing reciprocity in the parent–child relationship by helping children and mothers understand one another's perspectives and correcting distortions in their mental representations of themselves, each other, and their relationship; (2) improving emotion regulation in both children and mothers in order to reduce internalizing and externalizing behaviors; and (3) addressing both children's and mothers' posttraumatic stress symptoms by identifying trauma triggers, normalizing traumatic responses, and learning to respond realistically to new threats. The treatment described below illustrates the clinical application of these principles, highlighting the use of a dual attachment and trauma framework.

THE CRUZ FAMILY: A CASE STUDY OF THE RECIPROCAL IMPACT OF ATTACHMENT AND TRAUMA

Mrs. Cruz and her children were referred to our program by a friend who knew that she was a victim of domestic violence and that her children had witnessed the abuse. Mr. and Mrs. Cruz were both second-generation Mexican Americans whose grandparents had immigrated to the United States. Both parents spoke English in the home and considered themselves Hispanic Americans who where well acculturated to the United States. The therapist in this case was European American. Cultural issues, whether implicitly or explicitly articulated, are part of every clinical encounter. However, we do not refer to specific interventions addressing cultural values in this case because despite having different cultural backgrounds, the therapist and the mother had shared goals for treatment and there were no instances in which cultural differences appeared to interfere with treatment progress.

During the assessment period, Mrs. Cruz reported that, over a period of 6 months, her husband had yelled at, pushed, and slapped her several times when he was high on drugs and alcohol. Anthony was 18 months old and Maria was 3 years old when the violence began. Mrs. Cruz thought that Maria probably was less aware of her father's violence than Anthony because Maria usually was in day care when it occurred. In contrast, Anthony had witnessed nearly all of the domestic violence in the home. In the last and most severe episode, Anthony walked into the living room and saw his father looming over his mother with his hands around her throat. When Mr. Cruz saw Anthony watching from the doorway, he ran out of the house. After Mrs. Cruz called the police, Mr. Cruz was arrested and spent some time in jail. He also received substance abuse treatment. After a 1-year separation, during which he had had only phone contact with his children, Mr. Cruz begged his wife to let him return to the home, telling her that he was no longer using drugs or alcohol and that he would never raise a hand to her again. Mrs. Cruz was eager to have her family back together and accepted her husband back into their home. As promised, Mr. Cruz had remained clean and sober and had not been aggressive to her since their reunion. Mrs. Cruz reported that her husband was very apologetic and committed to repairing his relationship with his wife and children. Mrs. Cruz denied that she or her husband had ever maltreated or neglected the children, and there were no child protective service reports.

Anthony's Traumatic Stress Symptoms

Since witnessing his father's violence toward his mother, Anthony (age 3) had been having nightmares, had regressed to wetting his bed, had difficulty going to sleep, was easily distractible, and had become more aggressive toward his sister. He also had difficulty tolerating frustration. He repeatedly banged his head on the floor and cried when asked to gather his toys or end his play. Mrs. Cruz also reported that Anthony's speech was difficult to understand and seemed delayed in comparison to his peers. In the home, Anthony frequently showed fear of his father. For example, whenever Anthony saw his mother and father arguing about household issues, he would cry out, "Don't hurt my mommy!" Anthony otherwise avoided his father at home. The frequency and intensity of these responses led the clinician to make a diagnosis of PTSD.

Anthony's Attachment Relationships

As mentioned above, Anthony often appeared fearful for his mother's safety in the home. Mrs. Cruz reported that he was extremely protective and caring toward her. She recalled a time when she was upset and he reached out his hand to gently stroke her cheek, as though their roles were reversed and he was caring for her.

The observations made during the assessment were consistent with Mrs. Cruz's reports. In one session, Anthony used the toy cooking utensils to prepare a meal, fed his mother tenderly, and urged her to eat all her food. However, when it was time to clean up, Anthony suddenly fell to the floor and began sobbing inconsolably. His mother attempted to comfort him but he continued to cry for several minutes. Mrs. Cruz appeared unsure of how to console him. Later, during a brief separation from his mother, Anthony retreated to a corner of the playroom and sat on the floor with a sad expression on his face. He said softly, "Mommy" but showed no other signs of searching for her. Upon Mrs. Cruz's return to the room, he turned his back to her and ran to the pile of toys on the floor.

Although Anthony's intense distress during the clean-up episode clearly indicated problems with affect regulation, his inability to obtain comfort from his mother and his mother's inability to soothe him also suggested some dysregulation of the attachment–caregiving system. Anthony's play and separation–reunion behavior contained elements of controlling–caregiving, ambivalent, and avoidant patterns of attachment. His relationship with his father was not directly assessed, but it appeared from Mrs. Cruz's reports that Anthony was fearful and avoidant of him, suggesting possible disorganization of the child's attachment to his father as a result of the violence that Anthony had witnessed and the yearlong separation that followed. Bowlby (1973) described the highly avoidant behavior displayed by toddlers following prolonged separations from their primary caregivers as "detachment." Anthony may have been distancing himself from his father because he was experiencing both fear of and detachment from him.

Maria's Traumatic Stress Symptoms

Mrs. Cruz reported that, for the past year and a half, Maria (age 5) had had difficulty falling asleep at night, often woke up from nightmares, and was exhausted during the day. She was quick to startle and often seemed "on edge." She also was disrespectful and aggressive toward both her mother and father. Maria seemed to be experiencing increased arousal and possibly some reexperiencing of the violence, but she did not show signs of numbing or interference with her developmental momentum and did not receive a PTSD diagnosis.

Maria's Attachment Relationships

During her play session with her mother, Maria chose to play a board game, and she created her own set of rules for the game that she demanded her mother follow. She became angry at one point when her mother misunderstood her instructions. Mrs. Cruz joined her daughter's play but appeared somewhat passive and tired during the session.

During the separation and reunion episode, Maria did not appear distressed by her mother's departure from the room and continued to play with the toys, looking up briefly when her mother returned and demanding, "Sit down and play with me!" Maria appeared somewhat punitively controlling toward her mother, behavior that was consistent with Mrs. Cruz's description of her as obstinate and difficult to manage. From Mrs. Cruz's reports, Maria often was avoidant of her father in the home.

Mrs. Cruz's Trauma History and Posttraumatic Stress Symptoms

Mrs. Cruz reported that she had witnessed her own father physically abuse her mother throughout her childhood. She remembered one time when her father pushed her mother into some shelves, shattering her mother's treasured dishes inside. Mrs. Cruz said that she had married her husband at a young age to escape her abusive home. Although her marriage had been good for the first several years, her husband began to drink heavily after he lost his job and the domestic violence started soon after that. From the assessment, the clinician determined that Mrs. Cruz met criteria for PTSD. She experienced panic attacks in response to memories of the violence, had difficulty sleeping at night, and avoided any mention of domestic violence on the television or in the newspaper.

Mrs. Cruz's Attachment History

Mrs. Cruz described her father as absent and distant throughout her childhood. When he was present, he was often critical of her. She denied that her father had ever physically abused her, but she stated that he sometimes spanked her when she had "broken his rules." Mrs. Cruz's mother often worked long hours to support the family. She seemed timid when in the home and Mrs. Cruz described her as "unavailable." In contrast, Mrs. Cruz's relationship with her grandmother appeared close and loving. Mrs. Cruz had clear and loving memories of cooking with her grandmother in the kitchen and being soothed by her when she was ill.

Although Mrs. Cruz's state of mind regarding attachment was not formally assessed with the AAI, her presentation seemed consistent with that of "earned security" (Roisman, Padrón, Sroufe, & Egeland, 2002). She described her difficult childhood experiences coherently and in a balanced way, expressing understanding toward her parents and gratitude toward her grandmother, who was still living. It appeared that, for Mrs. Cruz, her grandmother was an "angel," willing and able to chase away the "ghosts" of parenting abuse and indifference when they appeared (Fraiberg, Adelson, & Shapiro, 1975; Lieberman, Padrón, Van Horn, & Harris, 2005). In working with traumatized families, an essential goal is to help parents identify beneficial influences in their pasts in order to help them draw on these benevolent figures to enhance their relationships with their children.

Mrs. Cruz's Caregiving Relationships with Her Children

Mrs. Cruz reported that she enjoyed being a mother, and that she had valued staying at home with her children to care for them. She reported that prior to the violence, she had spent hours each day playing with the children, taking them on outings to the park, and reading to them. While they continued to do some of these activities together, she felt that her children no longer listened to her and had become difficult to control. Mrs. Cruz reported that she often "walked away" from conflicts with her children because she felt overwhelmed by their disagreements.

At the end of the assessment, Mrs. Cruz reported, like many victims of domestic violence, that she had never before discussed her difficult life experiences with another person and that she felt relieved by being able to tell some of her life story to the clinician. The clinician assured Mrs. Cruz that her symptoms were expectable given her frightening experiences, provided information about PTSD, and reframed Mrs. Cruz's anxiety as an understandable response to her abusive experiences and to her fear that her husband might become violent again. Mrs. Cruz declined the clinician's offer of a referral for individual psychotherapy on the grounds that she had little spare time and no consistent child care. Nonetheless, after five individual meetings with the clinician during the assessment phase, Mrs. Cruz reported a decrease in her symptoms, suggesting that the assessment of a parent's functioning, within the context of a supportive relationship, can have positive intervention effects in itself.

An Attachment- and Trauma-Informed Case Formulation

The clinician drew on both attachment and trauma theory in her conceptualization of the Cruz family's struggles. The assessment suggested that, prior to the domestic violence, the children's relationships with their mother had been positive and their attachments to her may have been secure. The clinician hypothesized that the family's relationship difficulties were related to the children's fear of their father following the domestic violence and their mistrust in their mother's ability to protect them. Their mistrust was compounded by Mrs. Cruz's struggle to care for the children while suffering from her own traumatic stress symptoms. It appeared that, in response to Mrs. Cruz's helplessness and fear, the children were responding with controlling behavior. The clinician identified these mother–child relationship patterns as suggestive of disorganization of the attachment–caregiving system (Lyons-Ruth et al., 1999; Solomon & George, 1999). Anthony may have been experiencing more distress than his sister following the violence not only because he had witnessed more of the abuse, but also because he was younger and more dependent on his parents for his sense of safety in the world (Lieberman & Van Horn, 2005). These hypotheses guided the clinician's interventions during treatment.

Treatment Sessions

CPP is usually conducted in weekly home- or clinic-based sessions lasting approximately 1 hour. The clinician and Mrs. Cruz decided to meet in the clinic rather than in the family's home because although Mr. Cruz was supportive of the children receiving treatment, he chose not to be part of the therapy. The clinician and Mrs. Cruz agreed that the treatment would be conducted with both children simultaneously because both children were symptomatic and relatively close in age and developmental stage and because Mrs. Cruz had limited time available for treatment.

Mrs. Cruz, Anthony, and Maria attended 40 sessions of CPP over the course of 1 year. There were many facets to their treatment, and the clinician drew on psychoanalytic theory, social learning theory, cognitive-behavioral therapy, and other approaches using the integrative model of CPP (Lieberman & Van Horn, 2005). However, for the purposes of this discussion, we focus on those aspects of the treatment that highlight the interplay between attachment and trauma. In presenting the clinical vignettes, we explain how the use of a dual lens can elucidate clinical issues and guide specific interventions within the therapy.

On Knowing What You Are Not Supposed to Know . . .

Prior to beginning treatment, the clinician asked Mrs. Cruz what the children understood about why they were coming in for therapy. Mrs. Cruz responded that she had never talked to the children about the therapy, nor had she ever discussed their father's violence with them. She said, "They didn't know he went to jail for a month for hitting me. I told Anthony and Maria that their father had gone to visit friends and was going to be away for a while." However, when the clinician inquired further, Mrs. Cruz admitted that the children may have overheard her and Mr. Cruz talk about his incarceration after he returned home.

The clinician explained to Mrs. Cruz the importance of acknowledging the violence to her children and telling them that they would be coming to see someone to help them talk about the frightening things that they had seen at home. Mrs. Cruz asked the clinician to help her do this. At the first session with Maria, Anthony, and their mother, the clinician said, "Your mom is bringing you here because she knows that I'm someone who helps children and their parents with the scary things that happened to them and how they feel about them." Immediately, Maria asked, "Like when Daddy gets angry and I get scared?" The clinician replied, "Yes, like when your daddy gets angry and then you get scared." Anthony responded differently, saying, "My Daddy's home now. My Daddy came back." His mother said to the clinician, "He says that a lot—he still cries out for his father when he wakes from his nap." The clinician replied, "It seems like it's still hard for Anthony to believe that his father is really home." Turning to Anthony, she said: "Your dad was gone for a long time, but now he is home and he doesn't want to go away again."

Maria's quick acknowledgment of her father's anger and her own fear highlighted her always-present awareness of her father's violence, which was particularly notable because her mother believed that she had been sheltered from the frightening episodes. Even when violence stops, the emotional sequelae for children continue. The little girl's words suggested that even very young children can get relief from acknowledging the frightening events that bring them into treatment.

Anthony's response suggested that for this little boy, the separation from his father was an additional stressor that had yet to be acknowledged within the family. Perhaps for this reason, his trust in his father's return home was still tenuous. Anthony's words also highlighted the coexistence of longing and fear in his relationship with his father. Acknowledging the ambivalence that children may feel toward a violent caregiver helps to normalize their often confusing internal responses.

Mrs. Cruz's long-standing silence regarding the violence is common among battered mothers. Parents often deny the occurrence of violence either because of shame about the abuse, a desire to forget, or a hope that children will remain unaffected. For Mrs. Cruz, Anthony, and Maria, the domestic violence and Mr. Cruz's subsequent absence from the home had been the proverbial "elephants in the room," looming large but never acknowledged.

As Bowlby (1979) described in his seminal paper "On Knowing What You Are Not Supposed to Know and Feeling What You Are Not Supposed to Feel," the denial of a child's reality can have lasting harmful effects. When very young children witness frightening events, such as violence between their parents, the death of a loved one, or community violence, they rely on their attachment figures to help them make sense of their experiences and to help them cope with their feelings. Too often, though, the attachment figure is unable to assist the child in this process because he or she may be traumatized by the same event or may be responding to memories of past frightening experiences. Many of the parents who seek treatment for recent traumas have never talked with their children about other difficult life events such as a death or divorce. As a result, traumatic experiences often are layered upon one another silently and without acknowledgment. This can impair children's relationships with their caregivers and impede their recovery from trauma.

One of the primary goals of CPP for families who have experienced trauma is to enable them to "speak about the unspeakable." For very young children, this might be through play. For older children who have more developed language, talking about the traumatic event may be more appropriate.

Danger and Safety within the Attachment Relationship

The dual themes of danger and safety predominate in CPP with families who have experienced trauma. A prerequisite for treatment is the establishment of safety both in real life and in the therapeutic setting. Children who witness violence suffer a disruption of their "secure base" (Bowlby, 1969/1982) and distrust their caregiver's ability to keep them safe. Parents often are unaware of their children's lingering fear. The therapist's role is to name and normalize these fears while helping the parents to take effective actions to increase safety in the home.

In the case of the Cruz family, this intervention included regularly assessing Mrs. Cruz's feelings of security in her relationship and the creation of a safety plan for her and her children that Mrs. Cruz agreed to follow if she ever felt threatened by her husband again. For Anthony and Maria, however, the issue of safety was more complicated because their mother had decided to allow their previously violent father back into the home. Although their father was no longer aggressive and he was trying to repair his relationship with his wife and children, his past violence continued to shape the children's feelings and behavior. The therapist's role was to facilitate a discussion of the children's fears while helping them put them in the perspective of current safety to the extent that this was realistic and accurate.

In the second treatment session, the clinician addressed the children's fears by saying: "Your mommy brought you here so that you could talk about the scary things you saw, the times you saw your daddy hit your mommy," the clinician said. "You have scary memories, but it's also tricky because your mommy feels that your dad is safe now, and that is why he's living with you again." Mrs. Cruz said, "Daddy wouldn't be in the house if I didn't feel it was safe." Maria then said, "Sometimes daddy says scary things." The clinician asked the child about these "scary things," and Maria responded, "Sometimes he talks angry. It scares me when I hear mommy cry—I don't want mommy to get hurt." Her mother looked very sad. The clinician then asked Mrs. Cruz how she felt to hear this from her child, and she replied, "It's really hard to hear it, because my role is to protect them." Mrs. Cruz and the clinician then talked about how Mrs. Cruz might bring her husband into this discussion, and how, as a couple, they could find ways to reassure the children that, even though their parents sometimes argued, their home was now safe.

In this session, Mrs. Cruz showed great insightfulness regarding her children's reliance on her for protection from harm and fear. The clinician built on this insight to help Mrs. Cruz promote security within the children's attachment relationships with their parents, by acknowledging the past trauma and striving to provide them with a sense of safety regarding their future.

A Child's Helplessness: Linking to Past Trauma within the Attachment Relationship

As he had during the assessment, Anthony continued to have difficultly with transitions at home, at school, and in the therapeutic setting. For example, whenever it was time to end a treatment session, he immediately began to cry and threw himself on the ground, sobbing loudly. Mrs. Cruz appeared embarrassed and frustrated during these episodes. Exasperated, she would threaten to take away a favorite toy when they returned home. This usually failed to end Anthony's crying. In session 5, the clinician said to Anthony, "Saying good-bye is so hard for you. It makes you feel so upset." Anthony looked up at the clinician but said nothing. "It seems as though it's hard for him to leave places—home, here, even day care," the clinician observed to Mrs. Cruz. Mrs. Cruz said that he did get frustrated easily: "He likes to have things just so, like his carrots not touching his meat." The clinician said, "It seems as though he likes to have some control over things—that's natural for little kids—and especially for him, because things have not felt in control at home at times, right?" Mrs. Cruz said she had never thought about it that way before. The clinician suggested that they might help Anthony anticipate his good-byes by pointing out to him when their time was almost up. She also began bringing in a large timer to each session that allowed Anthony to see how much time was left in session. At home and at school, Mrs. Cruz made an effort to help talk with Anthony about transitions before they occurred, and his tantrums decreased substantially.

In this example, the clinician implemented a two-pronged intervention to help Anthony cope with the ending of sessions and other transitions in his life. First, she interpreted his difficulty with situations that felt out of his control—such as the ending of therapy sessions—as a reaction to the helplessness that he had felt witnessing the conflict and violence between his parents. This approach targeted Mrs. Cruz's negative attributions toward her son and reframed the child's behavior as an understandable response to his past frightening experiences with his attachment figures.

Mrs. Cruz then appeared more tolerant and understanding of her child, and this changed attitude in turn improved her ability to soothe him when he was distressed. Anthony's posttraumatic and disorganized symptoms decreased in tandem with the improvement in the quality of the parent–child relationship. The clinician also suggested concrete changes that Mrs. Cruz could make in helping Anthony anticipate transitions in the future, and she modeled effective action by bringing in a new clock that would appeal to a child at his developmental stage.

Understanding Children's Hypervigilance: Protecting the Attachment Figure

In session 10, Mrs. Cruz mentioned to the clinician that her children were having trouble getting ready for school on time in the mornings. The clinician learned that both children were still tired when they woke each day. When asked about the children's sleep schedule, Mrs. Cruz reported that she usually left the television on all night in the children's room and that the children stayed up late watching shows. The clinician asked what made it difficult for Mrs. Cruz to turn off the television and help the children get to sleep earlier. Mrs. Cruz was evasive and vague in her answers. Finally, the clinician asked, "I wonder if I'm pushing this issue too much? I sense that you're not sure what you'd like to do about the television." Mrs. Cruz said that she *was* unsure what to do about it. She added that it didn't matter what she did, because "the kids would just turn the television back on if I turned it off." The clinician commented, "Somehow, it seems that the children have a lot of control of how things go at bedtime. I wonder why that might be?" Mrs. Cruz suddenly paused and looked stricken. "I think," she said softly, "that the children watched television late at night because that was when we used to fight the most."

Turning to the children, the clinician said, "I know you worry about your mommy getting hurt. Your mommy and I are wondering if you stay up late at night because you're worried about her." Maria nodded her head. "When I close my eyes," she said, "I see monsters." Anthony then exclaimed, "Monster daddy!" Their mother looked upset and asked the therapist, "Are they saying that their daddy's a monster?" The clinician replied, "I think that the children are telling us that they remember what happened, and that they're still scared by it." Mrs. Cruz responded, "I didn't know all this. I didn't know that Maria didn't want to sleep because she was afraid." The clinician said, "I think the children know that you and their dad are trying to make their home safe for them, but they also are still worried that their dad might become violent again. I think they're looking for signs from you that they can relax and not worry so much. Maybe by turning off the TV and putting them to bed at an earlier hour you can help them learn that things are safer now." Mrs. Cruz responded with surprise and interest to this suggestion.

In this session, the clinician detected ambivalence and feelings of helplessness in Mrs. Cruz's approach to her children's bedtime routine. When traumatized mothers discuss their parenting, they often describe themselves as helpless and passive. Their children, in contrast, are either described as out of control and unmanageable or as extremely precocious and caring of the mother. These mothers seem to have abdicated caregiving of their children, and their children have inverted the parent–child role in response to this parenting vacuum (Lyons-Ruth et al., 1999; Solomon & George, 1999). When faced with evidence of this dysregulated attachment–caregiving pattern in the Cruz family, the clinician attempted to highlight for Mrs. Cruz her children's unresolved fear of their father, rooted in his past violence. At the same time, the clinician suggested to Mrs. Cruz ways that she might be able to provide structure and reassurance to decrease her own and her children's feelings of helplessness. Following this intervention, Mrs. Cruz was able to turn off the television at night, and she was surprised that the children went to bed without protest. The ease with which the children adapted to this new routine suggested that they actually may have been relieved and comforted when their mother finally set limits on their bedtime in order to foster their well-being.

Aggression within the Attachment Relationship: A Trauma Trigger for Mother

In session 17, Mrs. Cruz entered the therapy room with a frown on her face. She looked tired and pale. The children, in contrast, ran happily into the room and began to look for some of their favorite toys. Almost immediately, Mrs. Cruz began to complain that her daughter had been "bad" this week—Maria was defiant, controlling, and manipulative, she said. The clinician tried to explore this further and included the children in the discussion. She said, "Your mom seems upset about how things are going at home. She's telling me, Maria, that you aren't getting along very well and that she doesn't know what to do right now." Maria looked at the clinician briefly but continued to play with some toy trucks on the floor. Her mother said, "Maria, we're talking to you. Listen!" Maria suddenly looked up at her mother and raised her hand as though to strike her. Mrs. Cruz froze where she was sitting and said nothing. At that moment, Anthony walked near Maria, stepping on her shoe. Maria burst into tears and crawled into her mother's lap as though she were an infant seeking comfort. Mrs. Cruz held Maria and rocked her gently. Both mother and daughter seemed relieved. The clinician, sensing that mother and child had quickly moved on from their conflict, asked if they could return to what had been bothering them. She said, "I think something happened a few moments ago that is important to talk about. I wonder if Maria is crying, not because her foot was stepped on, but because of what happened between the two of you before that. It seemed like you were talking about how upset you were with Maria this week. And then you got angry with her when she didn't respond to my question. Then Maria got so angry and upset that she felt the urge to hit you." The little girl looked at the clinician and nodded, crawling deeper into her mother's lap. The clinician turned to the mother and both children and said, "But hitting people is wrong. Your daddy hit your mommy in the past, and that was very scary. Now it's scary for your mom to see Maria want to hit her, because she remembers that frightening time with your dad."

This interaction between Maria and Mrs. Cruz can be viewed through the dual lens of trauma and attachment theory. Examining it from the perspective of trauma, Maria's threatened violence toward her mother might be understood as identification with the aggressor, her father. Mrs. Cruz's frozen response suggested that Maria's raised hand may have triggered memories of her husband's violence. Attachment theory suggests that Maria was using violence as a way of exerting control in the face of her mother's helplessness, a pattern that would be consistent with the identified trajectory from infant disorganization to controlling behavior at school age (Solomon & George, 1999). The clinician used these hypotheses in attempting to intervene to break the negative cycle she observed between mother and child. She interpreted Mrs. Cruz's reaction as a traumatic stress response, making the link to the father's violence as a way of explaining it to the mother and her children. She acknowledged the daughter's anger and mother's fear, giving voice to their internal experiences. At the same time, the clinician modeled appropriate behavior for the mother by not ignoring her daughter's aggression and remaining helpless in the face of it, demonstrating that safety within attachment relationship comes from setting limits regarding violence.

Identifying Traumatic Reminders
within the Attachment Relationship

In session 20, Mrs. Cruz reported that Anthony had wet his bed the night before, which surprised her because he had not done this since the early weeks of treatment. The clinician asked Mrs. Cruz if anything had changed in their life recently that might have triggered this regression for Anthony. Mrs. Cruz thought for a while and said, "Well, my husband came home late from work last night—around 3:00 A.M.—because he's taken on a later shift at his job." With some questioning from the clinician, Mrs. Cruz explained that Mr. Cruz had been passing by the children's room when he saw Anthony standing up in bed, as though frozen there. The child stared at his father and began to urinate while standing on his bed. The clinician asked Mrs. Cruz if her husband had ever come home in the middle of the night before. Mrs. Cruz paused and said, "Yes. He used to leave the house after our fights and not return until very late at night." The clinician then suggested that, for Anthony, seeing his father return home in the middle of the night might have reminded him of other times that his father had come home late, after episodes of violence. His father's late return home could be a "traumatic reminder" for Anthony, the clinician explained. "I wonder," the clinician asked, "how we might help Anthony understand the difference between the present and the past?" Mrs. Cruz turned to Anthony, who was playing with a puzzle on the floor. She said, "I want you to know that Mommy and Daddy are not angry with each other now. Daddy came home late last night because he has a new job and he needs to work at night sometimes. But we are not fighting with each other." Anthony nodded his head but didn't say anything. Mrs. Cruz said to the clinician, "It's really hard to think about how much he might remember." The clinician nodded and said, "It must be difficult to realize this. I think we are learning that, although much of your conflict with their father was in the past, it is still feeling very present for the children."

Anthony's frozen posture and urination when he saw his father return home late at night appeared to be disorganized behavior, possibly resulting from Anthony's contradictory urges to approach his father for comfort and avoid his father because of fear. In this case, the attachment figure served as a traumatic reminder for the child. Mr. Cruz's late return home triggered Anthony's disorganized behavior, highlighting the potential overlap between posttraumatic stress responses and disorganization within the attachment relationship.

Children exposed to trauma may continue to be reminded of the frightening experience by cues in their environment. When these traumatic reminders remain unidentified by the caregiver, the child's sense of security is undermined because the child continues to feel fear, often unpredictably and without alleviation. Caregivers who fail to recognize and understand the meaning of the traumatic reminder also may unwittingly exacerbate the child's symptoms by rejecting or punishing the child (Lieberman & Amaya-Jackson, 2005). Once a traumatic reminder has been identified for a child, the most effective intervention is to remove the trigger from the child's environment. When this is not possible, the caregiver can gradually expose the child to the reminder in a safe and modulated way. With older children who have adequate language skills, the caregiver can help anticipate the occurrence of the traumatic reminder and help the child cope with resulting negative emotions. By talking about the nonviolent meaning of his father's late return home, Mrs. Cruz was helping Anthony gradually disassociate this experience from its previously frightening meaning.

Creating a Trauma Narrative
within the Attachment Relationship

One of the primary CPP therapeutic strategies is to help children and their parents construct a joint trauma narrative that weaves their often fragmented memories of the trauma into a fabric composed of events, cognitions, and emotions. The story may be told verbally or through play, depending on the child's developmental level and facility with expressive language. Play is used as a frequent port of entry because children often use play to depict their innermost experiences (Erikson, 1950; Slade, 1994).

In the Cruz family, Maria, at age 5, had begun to put her experience of her father's violence into words. After a few treatment sessions, she was able to talk about her fears "when Mommy hit Daddy" and about her memories of hearing her parents fighting in their room at night. Anthony, however, did not join in her storytelling until relatively late in the treatment. Only 3 years old, and having experienced some regression in his expressive language following the violence, Anthony gravitated toward toys rather than words to describe his experiences. His play at the start of treatment was quite constricted, focusing on building small towers with blocks or playing with small cars on the floor. There seemed to be little symbolic meaning in his play throughout the early stages of treatment.

Twenty-five sessions into treatment, Mrs. Cruz reported that she and her husband recently had been arguing at home, and that both children seemed upset by it. While Mrs. Cruz spoke, the children played on the floor, building an elaborate tower. Several minutes later, Anthony approached the wooden dollhouse in the corner of the playroom. He picked up a boy and a girl doll and placed them on two beds. The clinician commented that it looked as though the dolls were going to sleep. Anthony nodded seriously. He then picked up a male doll and a female adult doll and placed them downstairs, below the children's room. He began hitting the two dolls together forcefully, again and again, without any comment. The clinician said, "It looks like those dolls are really getting hurt. I wonder if you're showing us something that you've seen or heard before?" Anthony continued with the play, making the female doll shout, "Stop it, I hate you!" The clinician looked at Mrs. Cruz, who seemed distressed watching her son play. Maria was also watching her brother. She then entered into the play. She grabbed the father doll and placed him in a car that she then drove away. The clinician said, "I wonder if Anthony and Maria are telling us about a time that you and their father fought, and then their father left the house? And the children were upstairs in their room, listening to everything? It must have been scary for the children." Anthony said, "Daddy pushed and yelled at Mommy and I was scared." The clinician nodded and said, "It is so scary to see your daddy hit your mommy." Mrs. Cruz moved to comfort her son. She put her arms around him and then looked at her daughter and said, "Mommy and daddy did fight, and it was scary. And daddy went away to jail. But we are trying not to fight anymore. We don't want you to be scared anymore."

It was not until relatively late in the treatment that Anthony began to engage in storytelling about his frightening experiences. Children take their own time to develop and mature, and it is important for clinicians to respect their rhythms in spite of external pressures to "cure" them quickly. By providing toys that might serve as props for his narrative but also allowing Anthony to approach his frightening memories at his own pace, the clinician strove to meet Anthony at his own developmental stage while also trying to foster growth. Although Mrs. Cruz initially seemed to struggle watching her son play out the scene of violence, she eventually was able to engage in the narrative and provide comfort for her son. This may not have been possible for her at the start of the treatment, when she had seemed more avoidant of reminders of the violence.

Throughout the remainder of the treatment, Anthony continued to elaborate on the scenes of conflict and violence he had witnessed as a toddler. With the therapist, his mother, and at times, Maria, helping to put words to aspects of his play, Anthony constructed a narrative of his traumatic experiences. Over time, Anthony also added scenes of reunion and reconciliation between his father and the rest of the family, suggesting that he was creating a story not just of trauma but also of recovery.

A Good Good-Bye: Planning the End of a Close Relationship

For all clients involved in psychotherapy, but particularly for children and parents who have experienced trauma, a thoughtful termination of treatment is essential. For children and parents who have experienced separations from their caregivers, losses, or unexplained absences of important figures in their lives, ending relationships may be extremely painful. During the course of CPP, the clinician may acquire the role of surrogate attachment figure through the consistent focus on providing a haven of safety for the child and parent. The termination of treatment may be difficult for clients and clinician, but it also provides an opportunity to experience a "good good-bye." The clinician can convey that separations and loss can be acknowledged and anticipated, and that these experiences do not always mean a loss of love (Lieberman & Van Horn, 2005).

In session 30, the clinician reminded the family that they would be ending treatment in a few weeks. Mrs. Cruz turned to her children and said, "We've been coming here for almost a year, and now it's time to end—remember that we came here because we wanted help with some of the scary things that happened before?" Maria was drawing and Anthony was playing with Play-Doh. Both children nodded solemnly. The clinician added, "We've talked about how your daddy hit your mommy, and how both of you saw that happen." Maria replied, "Daddy said really mean things to mommy. But he doesn't say mean things anymore. He's a lot nicer now." The clinician replied, "Yes, your mom told me that your dad has made a lot of good changes, and he's safer now." Both children nodded. The clinician looked at Mrs. Cruz and said, "Your mom told me that she wanted your dad to come back and live with you, but only if he could be safe and not say and do such mean things. And it sounds like that has happened. Is that right, mom?" Mrs. Cruz said that was true. The clinician asked, "Do you feel as though things have worked out the way that you had hoped?" Mrs. Cruz replied, "Yes, it was the right choice. I didn't want my children to grow up without a father."

Shortly after this interaction, the clinician asked Mrs. Cruz how she felt about ending treatment. She said, "I've really benefited from coming here, and the children have, too." The clinician asked her what kinds of things had gotten better, and Mrs. Cruz explained, "I've been able to talk with them about what happened, about the scary things. I can talk to them now not only about the good things, but also about the bad things that happen, about good feelings and bad feelings. Also, last week the kids made a mess in the living room, and they dropped some glue on the floor. I would have reacted differently a year ago. I would have gotten really angry. Now I don't get upset about the small things. I keep them in proportion more."

Mrs. Cruz's words suggest that this was a successful treatment for her and her children. She no longer avoided discussing their father's violence with them, and she was now able to help them acknowledge both their positive and negative feelings toward her and her husband. She seemed to have gained insight into her past tendency to react quickly with anger to her children's misbehavior, and she felt more in control of her responses to them. Mrs. Cruz was no longer the helpless parent that she had appeared to be at the beginning of treatment; she was now more mindful and in control of how she cared for her children. A posttreatment assessment revealed that Mrs. Cruz no longer had a PTSD diagnosis and was experiencing minimal anxiety in her daily life. She also reported more pleasure in parenting and increased trust and collaboration with her husband.

The children's well-being, in turn, was significantly improved. Anthony no longer was wetting his bed at night, having tantrums at home or at school, being inappropriately aggressive with his sister, or showing fear of his father. His expressive language had improved considerably. His traumatic stress symptoms had improved to the point that he no longer met criteria for PTSD. In his final play and separation-reunion experience with his mother during the posttreatment assessment, Anthony was able to complete a complex puzzle with some help from his mother, and he was able to tolerate the frustration of having to end his play before he had completed his goal of building a tower out of blocks. When his mother left the room during the separation–reunion task, he noted her departure but actively engaged with toys until her return, when he welcomed her back into his play.

Maria also seemed to have benefited from the therapy with her mother and brother. Like her brother, she now went to bed at an early hour each night and she no longer saw "monsters" when she closed her eyes. She woke up rested and ready to start the day. She was less aggressive and controlling toward her mother and was more cooperative with her. In the separation–reunion episode at the end of treatment, Maria said good-bye to her mother when she left the room, and she included her mother in her gentle play with a baby doll when her mother returned.

OUTCOMES OF CHILD–PARENT PSYCHOTHERAPY: WHAT THE RESEARCH REVEALS

CPP appeared to have helped Maria, Anthony, and Mrs. Cruz decrease their trauma symptoms and improve their attachment and caregiving relationships. But are the results generalizable to other families? Research now has documented the benefits of this treatment approach for preschool children who have witnessed domestic violence and their mothers on a larger scale. Following 1 year of CPP, children displayed significantly fewer behavior problems and posttraumatic stress symptoms and diagnoses than children who received cases management and treatment as usual in the community. Their mothers also reported significantly less avoidance of traumatic memories related to the violence (Lieberman, Van Horn, & Ghosh Ippen, 2005). These outcomes were maintained 6 months after treatment ended (Lieberman, Ghosh Ippen, & Van Horn, 2006).

Although we are still analyzing data regarding treatment effects on the quality of child–parent relationships in this sample of preschoolers exposed to domestic violence, previous research suggests that CPP can benefit the attachment relationship. For example, in a sample of low-income Latina mother–infant dyads, infants receiving CPP displayed significantly less anxious attachment and significantly enhanced partnership with their mothers, compared to those in the nontreatment control group. Their mothers, in turn, showed higher levels of empathy and interactiveness with their children (Lieberman, Weston, & Pawl, 1991). CPP also has been shown to be effective in improving maltreated preschool children's attachment-related representations of themselves and their mothers, as well as their expectations of the mother–child relationship (Toth, Maughan, Manly, Spagnola, & Cicchetti, 2002). Finally, toddlers of depressed mothers who received CPP showed a significant increase in attachment security and a reduction in disorganized behavior with their mothers, compared to those in a nontreatment control group (Cicchetti, Toth, & Rogosch, 1999). Taken together, these findings suggest that CPP effectively integrates an attachment and trauma framework to help children and their parents recover from frightening life events.

SUMMARY AND CONCLUSIONS

In this chapter, we have proposed that the assessment and treatment of traumatized children should be conducted using a dual attachment and trauma framework. Traumatic experiences impact the quality of children's attachment relationships with their caregivers, and at the same time, children's attachment relationships can moderate the impact of trauma on their development. CPP is based on these principles, and on the resulting conclusion that children's recovery from trauma must take place within the context of their critical relationships with their caregivers.

The case of a child witnessing domestic violence highlights the interplay of attachment and trauma. Domestic violence directly challenges the child's trust that caregivers will be reliable protectors from harm. It also has frightening, potentially traumatizing effects on both the child and caregiver, which can lead to negative attributions, anger, and failure of the parent to respond to a child's cues for comfort and security. Any of these pathways can lead to a disorganized attachment relationship.

Domestic violence is but one example of a traumatic event that can derail a previously secure relationship between child and parent. Children rely on their caregivers to help them make sense of and regulate their emotional responses to all kinds of frightening events. Therefore, all traumatic experiences in young children's lives—whether the result of impersonal, external forces or acts perpetrated by the parent—have the potential to dysregulate the attachment system through their negative effects on individual family members and their relationship patterns (Lynch & Cicchetti, 2002). The negative impact of traumatic events on the family system can shed light on the elevated rates of disorganized attachment in high-risk populations (van IJzendoorn et al., 1999), where young children and their parents are more likely to be exposed to family violence, community violence, and other traumatic stressors. While consistent with Bowlby's (1969/1982) focus on the importance of real-life events in shaping attachment patterns, these findings suggest an

extension of Bowlby's attachment theory beyond the parent–child relationship to include other external stressors in the family's life. We pro-
pose that, by assessing trauma, child vulnerability, and the quality of the
attachment relationship, clinicians and researchers can build much-
needed bridges between trauma and attachment theory, incorporating
sustained clinical attention to the role of environmental factors in the etiology and perpetuation of a child's mental health problems (Lieberman,
2004; Lynch & Cicchetti, 2002; Pynoos et al., 1999).

In the case of the Cruz family, the clinician drew on research findings regarding disorganized attachment in infancy, controlling behavior
in preschool years, and parental helplessness to inform her assessment,
case conceptualization, and interventions during treatment. Attachment-
based research measures such as the Strange Situation and the AAI have
provided a wealth of empirical results with rich clinical implications, but
to date, there has been relatively little discussion about how these measures and their findings might be applied to clinical work. There is an
inherent tension between clinical work and research. Clinicians attempt
to understand the individual child as deeply and thoroughly as possible
in the context of his circumstances, using information about normal
development and developmental psychopathology to help the child. In
contrast, researchers aim to make generalizations across groups of children, using standardized assessments with precise approaches to mea-
surement and coding. Generalizations that apply to groups may or may
not be applicable to any one individual, with the result that the clinician
must be constantly on the lookout for confirmatory clinical evidence
when applying general principles to a particular child. At the more concrete level, both the Strange Situation and the AAI require intensive
training to learn their protocols and achieve coding reliability, and clinicians may not have the opportunity or inclination to do this training. In
addition, the Strange Situation relies on a highly structured series of
time-limited separation and reunion episodes; clinicians may feel that
this protocol is not appropriate to an unstructured therapeutic context.

In our own clinical research with children and parents, we have
used these measures to enhance our understanding of the quality of family relationships and the relational impact of trauma. However, we
believe that classifying children or adults according to their attachment
patterns is less important than identifying the psychological and interpersonal process that might lead a child to engage in avoidant, ambivalent, or disorganized behavior with a parent. All children may show
avoidance with a caregiver at some point; the question is where the

avoidance falls on a continuum from normal to disordered interaction patterns (Fraiberg, 1981/1987). Knowing the context of these behaviors is critical in understanding their meaning. Clinicians can play a valuable role in interpreting and contextualizing the information provided by the Strange Situation or AAI because they have a detailed knowledge of the child's individual characteristics and life circumstances, beyond the behavior elicited by a brief separation and reunion episode in the laboratory. If clinicians choose not to use structured attachment measures, they can still mine the rich literature on attachment, based on groups of children, to inform their approach to a particular child.

The case study of the Cruz family illustrates that the themes of attachment and trauma run throughout CPP for children who have witnessed domestic violence or other traumatic life events. Danger and safety, helplessness, protection, aggression, separation, and loss are simultaneously trauma and attachment themes, interwoven in the play and narratives of children who have had frightening experiences. Using both an attachment and trauma lens enables the clinician to make interventions that speak to both the frightening nature of children's experiences and the impact of these events on their relationships with their caregivers. In so doing, treatment addresses not only children's traumatization, but also their recovery.

REFERENCES

Ainsworth, M., Blehar, M., Waters, E., & Wall, S. (1978). *Patterns of attachment: A psychological study of the Strange Situation.* Hillsdale, NJ: Erlbaum.

American Psychiatric Association. (1994). *Diagnostic and statistical manual of mental disorders* (4th ed). Washington, DC: Author.

Belsky, J., & Fearon, R. M. P. (2002). Infant–mother attachment security, contextual risk, and early development: A moderational analysis. *Development and Psychopathology, 14,* 293–310.

Bowlby, J. (1973). *Attachment and loss: Vol. 2. Separation: Anxiety and anger.* New York: Basic Books.

Bowlby, J. (1979). On knowing what you are not supposed to know and feeling what you are not supposed to feel. *Canadian Journal of Psychiatry, 24*(5), 403–408.

Bowlby, J. (1982). *Attachment and loss: Vol. 1. Attachment.* New York: Basic Books. (Original work published 1969)

Busch, A., & Lieberman, A. F. (2006). *Maternal attachment representations predict children's IQ following exposure to domestic violence.* Manuscript in preparation.

Chemtob, C. M., & Carlson, J. G. (2004). Psychological effects of domestic violence on children and their mothers. *International Journal of Stress Management, 11*(3), 209–226.

Cicchetti, D., Toth, S. L., & Rogosch, F. A. (1999). The efficacy of toddler–parent psychotherapy to increase attachment security in offspring of depressed mothers. *Attachment and Human Development, 1*(1), 34–66.

Cohen, J. A., Mannarino, A. P., Berliner, L., & Deblinger, E. (2000). Trauma-focused cognitive behavioral therapy for children and adolescents: An empirical update. *Journal of Interpersonal Violence, 15*(11), 1202–1223.

Cook, A., Spinazzola, J., Ford, J., Lanktree, C., Blaustein, M., Cloitre, M., et al. (2005). Complex trauma in children and adolescents. *Psychiatric Annals, 35*(5), 390–398.

Crowell, J. A., Feldman, S. S., & Ginsberg, N. (1988). Assessment of mother–child interaction in preschoolers with behavior problems. *Journal of the American Academy of Child and Adolescent Psychiatry, 27*(3), 303–311.

Erikson, E. (1950). *Childhood and society.* New York: Norton.

Fraiberg, S. (1981/1987). Pathological defenses in infancy. In *Selected writings of Selma Fraiberg* (pp. 183–202). Columbus: Ohio State University Press.

Fraiberg, S., Adelson, E., & Shapiro, V. (1975). Ghosts in the nursery. *Journal of the American Academy of Child Psychiatry, 14,* 387–421.

Freud, S. (1955). Beyond the pleasure principle. In J. Strachey (Ed.), *The standard edition of the complete psychological works of Sigmund Freud* (Vol. 18). London: Hogarth Press. (Original work published 1920)

George, C., Kaplan, N., & Main, M. (1984, 1985, 1996). *Adult Attachment Interview Protocol.* Unpublished manuscript. University of California at Berkeley.

Hesse, E. (1999). The Adult Attachment Interview: Historical and current perspectives. In J. Cassidy & P. R. Shaver (Eds.), *Handbook of attachment: Theory, research, and clinical applications* (pp. 395–433). New York: Guilford Press.

Hesse, E., & Main, M. (2000). Disorganized infant, child, and adult attachment: Collapse in behavioral and attentional strategies. *Journal of the American Psychoanalytic Association, 48*(4), 1097–1127.

Koenen, K., Moffitt, T., Caspi, A., Taylor, A., & Purcell, S. (2003). Domestic violence is associated with environmental suppression of IQ in young children. *Development and Psychopathology, 15,* 297–311.

Lieberman, A. F. (2004). Traumatic stress and quality of attachment: Reality and internalization in disorders of infant mental health. *Journal of Infant Mental Health, 25*(4), 336–351.

Lieberman, A. F., & Amaya-Jackson, L. (2005). Reciprocal influences of attachment and trauma: Using a dual lens in the assessment and treatment of infants, toddlers, and preschoolers. In L. J. Berlin, Y. Ziv, L. Amaya-Jackson, & M. T. Greenberg (Eds.), *Enhancing early attachments: Theory, research, intervention, and policy* (pp. 100–124). New York: Guilford Press.

Lieberman, A. F., Ghosh Ippen, C., & Van Horn, P. (2006). Child–parent psychotherapy: 6-month follow-up of a randomized controlled trial. *Journal of the Academy of Child and Adolescent Psychiatry, 45*(8), 913–918.

Lieberman, A. F., Padrón, E., Van Horn, P., & Harris, W. (2005). Angels in the nursery: The intergenerational transmission of benevolent parental influences. *Infant Mental Health Journal, 26*(6), 504–520.

Lieberman, A. F., & Van Horn, P. (2005). *Don't hit my mommy!: A manual for child–parent psychotherapy with young witnesses of family violence.* Washington, DC: Zero to Three.

Lieberman, A. F., Van Horn, P., & Ghosh Ippen, C. (2005). Toward evidence-based treatment: Child–parent psychotherapy with preschoolers exposed to marital violence. *Journal of the American Academy of Child and Adolescent Psychiatry, 44*(12), 1241–1248.

Lieberman, A. F., Van Horn, P., & Ozer, E. J. (2005). Preschooler witnesses of marital violence: Predictors and mediators of child behavior problems. *Development and Psychopathology, 17*(2), 385–396.

Lieberman, A. F., Weston, D. R., & Pawl, J. H. (1991). Preventive intervention and outcome with anxiously attached dyads. *Child Development, 62*, 199–209.

Lynch, M., & Cicchetti, D. (2002). Links between community violence and the family system: Evidence from children's feelings of relatedness and perceptions of parent behavior. *Family Process, 41*(3), 519–532.

Lyons-Ruth, K., Bronfman, E., & Atwood, G. (1999). A relational diathesis model of hostile–helpless states of mind: Expressions in mother–infant interaction. In J. Solomon & C. C. George (Eds.), *Attachment disorganization* (pp. 189–212). New York: Guilford Press.

Lyons-Ruth, K., & Jacobvitz, D. (1999). Attachment disorganization: Unresolved loss, relational violence, and lapses in behavioral and attentional strategies. In J. Cassidy & P. R. Shaver (Eds.), *Handbook of attachment: Theory, research, and clinical applications* (pp. 520–554). New York: Guilford Press.

Main, M., & Cassidy, J. (1988). Categories of response to reunion with the parent at age 6: Predictable from infant attachment classifications and stable over a 1–month period. *Developmental Psychology, 24*(3), 415–426.

Moss, E., St-Laurent, D., & Parent, S. (1999). Disorganized attachment and developmental risk at school age. In J. Solomon & C. C. George (Eds.), *Attachment disorganization* (pp. 160–186). New York: Guilford Press.

Osofsky, J. (2003). Prevalence of children's exposure to marital violence and child maltreatment: Implications for prevention and intervention. *Clinical Child and Family Psychology Review, 6*(3), 161–170.

Pynoos, R. S., Steinberg, A. M., & Piacentini, J. C. (1999). A developmental psychopathology model of childhood traumatic stress and intersection with anxiety disorders. *Biological Psychiatry, 46*, 1542–1554.

Roisman, G. I., Padrón, E., Sroufe, L. A., & Egeland, B. (2002). Earned-secure attachment status in retrospect and prospect. *Child Development, 73*(4), 1204–1219.

Scheeringa, M. S., & Zeanah, C. H. (1995). Symptom expression and trauma variables in children under 48 months of age. *Infant Mental Health Journal, 16*(4), 259–270.

Schuder, M., & Lyons-Ruth, K. (2004). "Hidden trauma" in infancy: Attachment, fearful arousal, and early dysfunction of the stress response system.

In J. D. Osofsky (Ed.), *Young children and trauma: Intervention and treatment* (pp. 69–104). New York: Guilford Press.

Schuengel, C., Bakermans-Kranenburg, M. J., & Van IJzendoorn, M. H. (1999). Frightening maternal behavior linking unresolved loss and disorganized infant attachment. *Journal of Consulting and Clinical Psychology, 67*(1), 54–63.

Slade, A. (1994). Making meaning and making believe: Their role in the clinical process. In A. Slade and D. P. Wolf (Eds.), *Children at play: Clinical and developmental approaches to meaning and representation* (pp. 81–107). New York: Oxford University Press.

Solomon, J., & George, C. C. (1999). The place of disorganization in attachment theory: Linking classic observations with contemporary findings. In J. Solomon & C. George (Eds.), *Attachment disorganization* (pp. 3–32). New York: Guilford Press.

Stamper, J., & Lieberman, A. F. (2006). *Traumatic stress symptoms and cognitive performance in preschoolers exposed to domestic violence.* Manuscript in preparation.

Toth, S. L., & Cicchetti, D. (1996). Patterns of relatedness, depressive symptomatology, and perceived competence in maltreated children. *Journal of Consulting and Clinical Psychology, 64*, 32–41.

Toth, S. L., Maughan, A., Manly, J. T., Spagnola, M., & Cicchetti, D. (2002). The relative efficacy of two interventions in altering maltreated preschool children's representational models: Implications for attachment theory. *Development and Psychopathology, 14*(4), 877–908.

van IJzendoorn, M. H., Schuengel, C., & Bakermans-Kranenburg, M. J. (1999). Disorganized attachment in early childhood: Meta-analysis of precursors, concomitants, and sequelae. *Development and Psychopathology, 11*(2), 225–249.

Zeanah, C. H., Danis, B., Hirshberg, L., Benoit, D., Miller, D., & Heller, S. S. (1999). Disorganized attachment associated with partner violence: A research note. *Infant Mental Health Journal, 20*(1), 77–86.

Zero to Three/National Center for Clinical Infant Programs. (2005). *Diagnostic classification of mental health and developmental disorders of infancy and early childhood* (rev. ed.). Washington, DC: Author.

CHAPTER SEVEN

The Circle of Security Project

A Case Study—"It Hurts to Give
That Which You Did Not Receive"

BERT POWELL, GLEN COOPER, KENT HOFFMAN,
and ROBERT MARVIN

The Circle of Security (COS) Project is an early-intervention program designed to alter the developmental pathway of at-risk parents and their young children (Hoffman, Marvin, Cooper, & Powell, 2006; Marvin, Cooper, Hoffman, & Powell, 2002). The focus of the intervention is to help caregivers reevaluate the accuracy of their internal representations of child and self when their child needs them for secure base/safe haven caregiving. Caregiver representations are the focus of the intervention because converging data support the notion that the state of mind of the caregiver organizes and directs caregiving behaviors, which in turn affects the child's security of attachment (Fonagy, Steele, & Steele, 1991). Prior to being involved in the intervention, many of the participants had a history of asking Head Start staff for specific behavioral suggestions, resulting in little change. We focus on the parent because of the conviction that the adult has more ability to change the relationship than the child, especially considering that all the children in this program are under the age of 5. The children are involved during the assessment videotapings, which take place preintervention, about two-thirds of the way through the intervention, and postintervention. The teachers and family service coordinators at Head Start participate in the protocol as support for the families and give the parents COS-informed feedback in their daily interactions with their children.

In this chapter, we describe the COS protocol and the therapeutic experience of one of the participants. She is a 19-year-old mother whom we will call Shelly. Her son's Head Start teacher referred Shelly to the COS intervention program because of her son's aggressive behavior in the classroom. Her son, whom we will call Jacob, was 3½ years old at the time of the referral. Shelly also reported difficulty managing Jacob's behavior in the home. Jacob's father lived out of the city and was not involved with the family.

CIRCLE OF SECURITY INTERVENTION

At the core of the intervention is the notion that insecure children have learned to divert ("miscue") their caregivers away from their basic attachment needs because cueing about their needs directly evokes distressful emotional states in their parents. When distressed, the parents' availability decreases. The children learn to optimize their connection to their parents by developing behavioral strategies that mask or exaggerate basic attachment needs, thus diminishing their parent's distress and gaining as much psychological proximity as possible.

The COS graphic (Figure 7.1) is used as a map to help parents understand attachment theory. The graphic facilitates parents' capacity to see the perpetual rhythm of how their children look to them for signals that it is okay to seek physical and psychological proximity as needed; "fill their emotional cups"; transition from attachment to exploration; look to them for signals that it is okay to explore; and explore their environment using parental support. The term "top half" represents the child's needs while using the parent as a secure base for exploration, while "bottom half" represents the child's needs when using the parent as a safe haven.

Parents are encouraged to be "bigger, stronger, wiser, and kind" and this function is called providing the "hands" on the circle. In the more troubled dyads when parents try to be "bigger and stronger" they

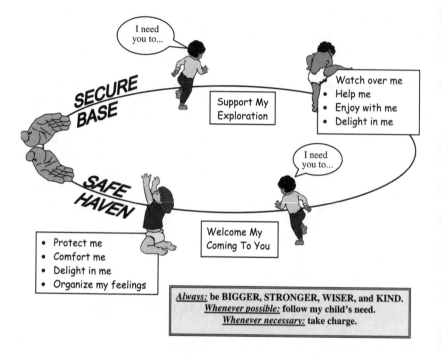

FIGURE 7.1. Circle of Security graphic: Parent attending to the child's needs. Copyright 2000 by Glen Cooper, Kent Hoffman, Robert Marvin, and Bert Powell.

sacrifice "kind" and become mean, or when they try to be "kind" they sacrifice "bigger and stronger" and become overly accommodating, allowing their children to be "in charge" of the relationship. Wisdom is the knowledge of how to be simultaneously bigger, stronger, and kind, as their children need them "all around the circle."

Children's insecure attachment strategies are a defensive solution to the problem that there is a deficit in at least one of the three basic caregiving functions of providing a secure base, a safe haven, or "hands." Participants are asked to look at video vignettes of parent–child interaction while answering a central question, "Does this behavior represent a 'top half' need, a 'bottom half' need, or a 'hands' need on the Circle?" By having the caregiver become more skilled at identifying children's needs on the Circle, a foundation of observational skills is developed that facilitates the parent seeing both secure and insecure attachment patterns in the relationship.

A key insecure parent–child interaction is selected from the video-tape of the preintervention Strange Situation Procedure (SSP) to review as the linchpin focus for change. The parents are encouraged to reevaluate their own insecure emotional state and internal representations of self and other evoked by their child's attachment behaviors. As parents change vital aspects of their caregiving during the program, many report both positive feelings of success and painful feelings as they begin to give their child that which was not given to them in their own early years. It takes courage and commitment by the parents to manage painful memories and a sense of loss while focusing on giving new dimensions of emotional security to their children. Each parent participates in three highly structured videotape reviews, watching selected clips from the parent–child assessments. Each video review has a unique focus with Phase 1 review focusing on parent's hidden strengths, Phase 2 focusing on the insecure linchpin interaction, and Phase 3 focusing on reinforcing emerging capacities. We discuss the COS intervention in more detail next.

Groups of six parents meet for 1 hour and 15 minutes a week for 20 weeks to focus on enhancing the attachment–caregiving aspects of their relationship with their children. Each caregiver and his or her child participate in an SSP before and within 10 days after the group intervention. For diagnostic purposes, a brief reading and cleanup episode was added at the conclusion of the standard SSP. The SSP was classified using Ainsworth's classification system for infants (Ainsworth, Blehar, Waters, & Wall, 1978) or the Preschool Attachment Classification System (Cassidy & Marvin, 1992).

Following the Strange Situation, the caregivers participated in the Circle of Security Interview (COSI; Cooper, Hoffman, Marvin, & Powell, 1997). This interview consists of questions regarding the parent's experience during the SSP, selected questions from the Parent Development Interview that focus on describing the relationship with the child (Aber, Slade, Cohen, & Meyer, 1989), and selected questions from the Adult Attachment Interview that focus on perceptions of how their own attachment history affects current parenting (George, Kaplan, & Main, 1985). The COSI is videotaped and lasts approximately 1 hour.

Every week for 20 weeks parents gather to discuss videotaped attachment–caregiving interactions between themselves and their children edited from the preintervention SSP and a modified SSP administered in the last half of the program. The COS graphic described above (Figure 7.1) is used as a map to help parents understand secure base/safe haven needs in their child. The video clips reviewed by parents are carefully selected to help them develop a specific interactional pattern that will enhance the security of their relationship with their child.

A framework for understanding secure and insecure states of mind regarding attachment (George, Kaplan, & Main, 1985) is introduced in week 9 of the program using the concept of "Shark Music" (see below). According to attachment theory parents learn a state of mind regarding their own attachment needs while growing up and tend to see their own child's needs through the same lens. Lyons-Ruth termed this learning "implicit relational knowing" and described these caregiving–attachment behaviors as rule-based procedures learned experientially and organized with or without language. Attachment is also a procedure that is learned prior to the development of language, based on "procedural memory," and represents "implicit relational knowing" (Lyons-Ruth et al., 1998) regarding specific ways to be with a caregiver during times of need.

In the COS parents learn about the concept of state of mind by contrasting one video clip set to two different kinds of music. This is termed "Shark Music." The video clip is of a scenic coastline and rain-forest. The first viewing is set to soft, serene music. The group members discuss the wonderful feelings this activates. The second viewing of the clip is set to a modified version of the soundtrack from *Jaws*. Discussing how this time they experience agitation and anxiety, the parents come to understand how much their own subjective experiences can affect their perceptions. Music is a good metaphor to help parents learn about state of mind because it evokes feeling and is not language based. Once parents grasp this concept they are asked what music they hear when their child has each of the needs described on the COS. Do they hear soothing music or "Shark Music"? The term "Shark Music" is a frequently used icon in the intervention describing the insecure implicit relational knowledge that must change in the parent in order for the child to be more secure.

From the inception of the COS project, a core goal has been to increase parents' reflective functioning, especially in regard to "Shark Music" (Fonagy, Steele, Steele, & Target 1997). Fonagy and colleagues have used the concept of reflective functioning to summarize a number of mental functions described in the literature under such terms as mentalization, theory of mind, metacognition, intentional stance, and observing ego. Our working definition for reflective functioning is "the psychological capacity for understanding one's own mental states, thoughts, feelings, and intentions as well as those of the other." Fonagy and colleagues (1991) showed that the reflective functioning of pregnant women predicted their child's attachment classification at 1 year of age. In addition, Fonagy, Steele, Steele, Higgit, and Target (1994) found that adults with high reflective functioning were able to transcend a deprived background and promote attachment security in their children.

CORE SENSITIVITIES

John Bowlby hypothesized that attachment relationships in early life become the building blocks for the creation of an "internal working model" that is used as a map to understand current and future relationships. Unfortunately, the richness of this concept was not expanded and clarified in his writing. In the field of object relations, there is an abundance of complex intrapsychic models that can be used to enrich the internal working model concept. If the internal working model is the lens through which interactions are interpreted then having a way to clinically describe the vicissitudes of different models is important for effective intervention, particularly if the focus of the intervention is to reevaluate inaccurate internal representations of self and child. The term "core sensitivity" was created to focus on the central emotional struggle for three prevalent working models (Masterson & Klein, 1995), with the objective of making the labels "experience near" (Kohut, 1971). The three core sensitivities are separation sensitive, esteem sensitive, and safety sensitive.

Core sensitivities are hypothesized to be an integral part of personality structure and tend to remain stable from one relationship to the next. In a sense, they are the perceived, yet unspoken rules and requirements that one believes must be followed in order to avoid the experience of abandonment. Intense need for connection and fear of the loss of connection are central organizing processes in the development of personality structure (Masterson, 1976). These core sensitivities are the basis of a parent's internal defensive process, which in turn often drives problematic parent–child interaction. Clarification of this process can inform and shape clinical interventions.

Even though these rules are amenable to change, they tend to be imposed on other relationships throughout a person's life. To help clarify the core sensitivities that organize parents' patterns of attachment–caregiving interaction, Cooper, Hoffman, and Powell (1998) have applied the object relations work of Masterson and Klein (e.g., 1995), Heinz

Kohut (e.g., 1971), and Otto Kernberg (e.g., 1975) to early childhood intervention. The COS assessment of core sensitivity is done while watching the standardized COSI (Cooper et al., 1997).

To clarify that we are referring to defensive strategies rather than personality disorders, and to make our terminology less confusing and pejorative for clinicians, we have shifted from the DSM-IV personality disorder terminology. We label the three basic patterns or sensitivities in the following way: separation sensitive (which in a rigid and pervasive form is borderline personality disorder); esteem sensitive (which in a rigid and pervasive form is narcissistic personality disorder); and safety sensitive (which in a rigid and pervasive form is schizoid personality disorder) (Hoffman, Cooper, Marvin, & Powell, 1997; Masterson & Klein, 1995). The sensitivities form a continuum from flexible and adaptive defensive strategies to rigid and pervasive personality styles. It is more difficult to discern the core sensitivity of a person who is on the flexible and adaptive end of the continuum than it is to discern the core sensitivity of one who is on the rigid and pervasive end. Fortunately for the purpose of treatment, the more flexible and adaptive people are, the less vital it is to identify their core sensitivity. The following is a thumbnail sketch to help clarify the nature of these sensitivities.

- Separation-sensitive parents have come to believe that to avoid abandonment, they must focus on what others want, need, and feel, while disavowing their own wants, needs, and feelings. The underlying belief is that if they act on their own behalf, they will be abandoned by those they most need.

- Esteem-sensitive parents have come to believe that who they are is not enough to be valued. Therefore, to protect themselves from abandonment they must prove that they are special through performing, achieving and acquiring the acknowledgment of others.

- Safety-sensitive parents have learned that the cost of being connected in a relationship is to give up having a self and to be controlled by the other. Therefore, the only way to have an intact sense of self is to be isolated. Since both being close and being isolated are ultimately unbearable, safety-sensitive individuals are constantly seeking a compromise between the two. However, this compromise keeps them in "limbo," neither actually in nor out of relationship. The safety sensitive individual lives in the dilemma of this nether land of unfulfilling relationships.

CASE PRESENTATION

The remainder of this chapter focuses on the experience of one COS participant, Shelly, with relevant theory inserted as needed. During the initial screening interview, Shelly presented as shy and uncertain. She stated that she wanted help managing Jacob's aggression and appeared passive and helpless about her role as a parent. The purpose of the screening interview was to determine if she had interest in learning about her relationship with Jacob, had even modest reflective functioning (Fonagy et al., 1997), and was capable of making the commitment to regularly attend a 75-minute COS group once a week for 20 weeks. Shelly met all three criteria and enrolled as a participant in the project.

The first step for Shelly in the COS project was to take part in a preintervention assessment. Since Jacob was 3½ years old the parent–child relationship was assessed using the Cassidy/Marvin Preschool SSP with a reading episode and a cleanup episode added at the end. The SSP is used both for research purposes, to assess the pre- and postattachment classification of the child, and for treatment purposes to organize the intervention by clarifying the strengths and struggles in the three COS domains of "secure base," "safe haven," and "hands" (Figure 7.1; Marvin et al., 2002). The COSI is used to assess both the parent's state of mind regarding the relationship with the child and his or her core sensitivity. Information from the SSP about the caregiver–child interaction and information from the COSI about the parent's state of mind regarding the child and about his or her core sensitivity is organized into a relationship-based treatment plan and a strategy for intervention.

During the 21-minute SSP there were numerous times Jacob's exploratory behaviors and his corresponding needs (i.e., the "top half" of the Circle) generated distress in his relationship with his mother. When they first entered the room, Jacob explored the toys as Shelly sat in a chair. Shelly immediately asked, "Do you want me to play with you?" and he quickly replied, "No." She acted as if she was not affected by his refusal, but her overly cheerful voice tone combined with an underlying look of rejection indicated otherwise. Acting overly happy in the face of distress is a defense termed *overbright* and this defense conveyed a mixed message to Jacob. Shelly then asked, "OK, you want me to sit here and watch?" to which Jacob answered, "Yes." Again, Mom said, "OK" with the same overbright demeanor. Shelly waited 6 seconds and then asked her son, "Do you want to read a book?" and he replied, "No." Once more, with an overbright tone attempting to hide her pain,

she proclaimed, "OK, I will just let you play." Jacob then began a mono-
logue concerning what he was doing, not actually speaking to his
mother. Shelly found this to be an opportunity to interact further with
her son. Within 20 seconds, she was with him on the floor trying to join
in his play. As Shelly pursued him, he turned his back to her. The interaction continued with his mother seeking involvement and Jacob trying to
play alone. Sometimes he answered his mother's questions and sometimes he ignored them. There were instances in which he joined his
mother for a few moments of positive play but these invariably ended
with his wanting to play on his own. Despite Shelly acting as if his interest in playing without her was acceptable, it was clear that she was hurt.
The relationship appeared to have developed a painful pattern in which
Jacob was continually fighting for independence and Shelly was fighting
for involvement. Shelly was not able to watch her son play and feel a
sense of joy, delight, and connection.

When Jacob was alone in the room, he proceeded with his play and
was only able to reveal his distress regarding the absence of his mother
in subtle ways. His lifeless play with the toys and his flat affect stood in
contrast to his animated play when Shelly was in the room. During one
brief but significant moment during her absence, he looked directly at
the one-way glass, behind which his mother was standing, with what
appeared to be a searching, longing glance. When his mother was
absent, he worked to maintain a facade that he was fine and simply playing with the toys. It was becoming obvious that Jacob had apparently
learned to minimize showing his experience of distress in a direct
fashion.

The manner in which a parent and child verbally and nonverbally
negotiate their "interactional dance" in the first few minutes of a
reunion reveals their core caregiving–attachment strategy (Ainsworth et
al., 1978; Cassidy & Marvin, 1992). When Shelly returned to the room
her first words were "What are you doing?" Jacob responded by playing
with his back to her and ignoring her until she asked a second time,
prompting him for a reply. In response to his mother's plea for a
response, he answered, "Nothing" while shrugging his shoulders and
keeping his back to her. Shelly then moved toward her son, sitting down
on the floor to be with him and trying to join in his play. When she
touched a toy, he protested and she said with her overbright voice, "OK,
I will just watch." After a couple of seconds Shelly asked, "Can I do this
one?" while she touched a toy, and Jacob said, "No." Shelly stood up,
saying, "I will leave you alone," and moved toward the chair with a

dejected demeanor. Jacob immediately called her back and directed her to "do this one." Shelly joined in the play for a few moments and then sat in the chair. As soon as she moved away, Jacob moved closer to her and simultaneously turned his back to her.

Within the terminology of attachment theory Jacob showed both avoidance and role reversal during the reunions. Role reversal describes the child taking a parental or organizing role because the parent abdicates a crucial parenting function. Role reversal is associated with disorganized attachment and negative developmental outcomes (Liotti, 1992; Main & Hesse, 1990; Sroufe, Egeland, Carlson, & Collins, 2005; van IJzendoorn, Schuengel, & Bakermans-Kranenburg, 1999). When a child is separated from a primary caregiver during the SSP his or her attachment behavioral system is activated. Given his flattened affect and searching looks into the one-way mirror, this was clearly the case with Jacob. However, when his mother returned to the room and was accessible he acted as if he did not need her and become both rejecting and controlling. Upon reunion, Jacob directed his mother as opposed to his mother helping him with his distress. Even though it appeared that he did not need her, as soon as she withdrew from him he told her to return. He needed her to be available while simultaneously seeking to be in control of their interaction, all the while acting as if he did not need her. Throughout much of the procedure, Shelly attempted to hide her pain. She accommodated to his direction and control, looking childlike and helpless in the interaction.

From the COS perspective, Shelly was struggling with the "top half of the Circle," the "bottom half of the Circle," and with providing "hands." Struggling with the top half of the Circle was demonstrated by her interfering with Jacob's exploration thus not adequately providing him with a secure base from which to explore autonomously. She was struggling with the bottom half of the Circle in that she was not effectively providing him with comfort and organizing his feelings when he was upset and needed her as a safe haven. She was not providing the guidance of "hands": taking charge when Jacob needed her to do so in a "bigger, stronger, wiser, and kind" manner (Figure 7.1).

Jacob's attachment behaviors had elements of multiple strategies. He showed resistance–ambivalence by pulling her in closer and pushing her away. He showed avoidance and ignoring by turning his back to her and pretending that he did not need her when he clearly did. He exhibited a controlling strategy by instructing his mother on what to do and directing her behavior in the reunions. No single pattern was predominant. Therefore, his SSP classification was insecure-other. In Cassidy and Marvin's preschool system, this classification indicates a mixture of contradictory, non-normative attachment patterns and for research purposes is regarded as a disturbed pattern with the same developmental trajectory as disorganized attachment. Parents with children classified as insecure-other are often more challenging to help than parents who have children classified as disorganized. Because multiple insecure patterns are used, a single insecure pattern cannot be selected as the linchpin for intervention. Thus, several patterns must be addressed, which in turn tends to make the treatment more complex.

When the time came for Shelly to get Jacob to pick up the toys, she pleaded with him as he resisted her timid directives, thus abdicating her role as the parent "in charge." However, there was one crucial moment that stood in contradiction to all other moments. When Shelly told Jacob, in a firm adult tone, to take a dirty toy out of his mouth, he promptly complied. This moment demonstrated what we call an "underused capacity." If a parent can do it once, she obviously has the skill and potential to do it again. Therefore, it is a potential strength the parent has in her behavioral repertoire, one that for defensive reasons is not being used on a frequent basis. Shelly was avoiding being in charge and providing leadership in moments when Jacob desperately needed her to do so. Within the COS framework, it is hypothesized that the caregiver is avoiding using this capacity because it evokes a feeling state ("Shark Music") that he or she does not want to reexperience. This makes the central focus of the intervention helping Shelly to reevaluate her state of mind when Jacob needs her and learning about how she protects herself from vulnerable emotions by abdicating her parental, "in charge" role. This differs significantly from the more traditional goal within many parenting programs where the focus is upon learning new skills.

During the COSI, which immediately proceeds the SSP, Shelly appeared confused by the questions. She thought her child did not need her during the SSP and reported feeling frightened when she was asked to leave her son during the separation because she anticipated that he would throw a temper tantrum. When asked to focus on herself and describe her own thoughts and feelings, she became anxious and frequently responded with the phrase "I don't know." At one point in the interview, she revealed that when Jacob had recently told her he loved her it was a real booster for her to know that someone "actually" loved her. This last statement poignantly revealed her insecurity about feeling cared for, while simultaneously indicating that she experienced emotional bonds as fragile.

Shelly's linchpin struggle was clarified by her answer to the question concerning what gives her the most pain in her relationship with Jacob. She responded, "Discipline," and then offered an instance of refusing to meet his demand for ice cream for breakfast. She stated, "I got mad at myself because I just made my son hate me, not like me, because I did not give him what he wanted." Her son's disapproval was profoundly distressing to Shelly because she felt that what was at stake was whether she was loved or not loved. Within her emotional worldview, if her son does not love her, he will abandon her. This makes Jacob's availability an essential ingredient in Shelly's emotional stability and gives 3-year-old Jacob a power over his mother that threatens not only her sense of security, but his as well. Her need for her son's availability creates a role-reversed relationship in which Jacob is forced to survive psychologically without a bigger, stronger, wiser, and kind mother to meet his needs. In COS language she is not adequately providing the "hands" on the Circle that he needs in order to experience either a secure base or a safe haven.

Shelly continued to talk about the ice cream incident. "But then I think, if I give him everything he wants, when he is not given what he wants he will act out and who knows what he could do." She recognized that if she inevitably gave her son what he wanted it would be harmful to him. Her capacity to have a realistic perspective regarding the consequences of her actions on her son is seen as a hidden strength. Shelly was, in that moment, showing that she had access to at least moderate levels of reflective functioning. Even though she did not consistently use her reflections to guide her behavior, it is far easier to help a parent learn to use existing reflective capacity than it is to forge a new capacity from a context of no previous experience in this area.

Shelly recognized what she needed to do, but it frightened her for reasons that had little to do with her 3-year-old son. Shelly's "ghosts in the nursery" (Fraiberg, Adelson, & Shapiro, 1975) were clearly haunting her capacity to parent Jacob. Seen within the context of "implicit relational knowing," Shelly was employing an insecure caregiving procedure with her son that was organized below the level of awareness, what Christopher Bollas (1987) calls the "unthought known." She knew she had anxious feelings when she tried to take charge, and realized that she could avoid them by accommodating to her son's demands. This process was "unthought" in that she had no language, no symbolic process to describe the meaning behind her feelings. She did not cognitively know why such fear was associated with the everyday act of setting limits and managing her child's anger. She simply knew fear and the preverbally learned protective procedure of avoiding conflict in order to make it go away.

Even though it takes going through the entire COSI to form a hypothesis regarding the parent's core sensitivity, the information offered the reader thus far is sufficient to formulate an initial impression. Because Shelly intensely required Jacob to care for her and include her in their interactions, safety sensitivity is not a likely option. A person who is safety sensitive tends to keep his or her child focused away from the relationship and seeks to promote self-sufficiency in the child. Parents who are safety sensitive are more comfortable when their children are on the "top half" of the Circle as opposed to the "bottom half." This was clearly not the case with Shelly.

The process of determining a parent's core sensitivity is facilitated by asking oneself differential questions while watching the tape of the COSI. These questions are designed to parse the meaning of the information from the COSI into one of the three categories. Examples of differential questions are:

1. Why does Jacob's acting as if he does not need Shelly have such emotional power over her?
   - Does it make her feel alone, helpless, and abandoned (separation sensitive)?
   - Does it make her rejected and a failure (esteem sensitive)?
2. What is the meaning behind Shelly's intrusion into her son's exploration?
   - Is she interfering to teach him to perform better so that she will appear and feel successful as a parent (esteem sensitive)?
   - Is she threatened by his autonomy because he will no longer need her and she will feel painfully alone and unwanted (separation sensitive)?

While these questions oversimplify the process, by asking them the therapist can begin to organize the meaning behind the parent's behavior and discourse, thus formulating a hypothesis regarding the parent's core sensitivity.

Shelly's core sensitivity was about separation. For her, Jacob initiating autonomy was the first step in a cascading process toward abandonment that would ultimately lead her to feeling alone, unloved, and unlovable. This matches with Shelly's history of feeling depressed, emotionally abandoned, and alone as a child. She hoped Jacob would protect her from these feelings by unremittingly loving her and never leaving her. For example, during the COSI when asked if she felt Jacob came into her life for a reason she stated that prior to becoming pregnant with him she was so depressed she did not want to live and he gave her a reason to go forward with her life. Later she stated there was nothing she wanted to repeat with Jacob that she learned from her mother because she did not feel "cared for" in the course of her own development.

Once the key issue in the parent–child interaction is identified, a video clip that most clearly shows the problem is selected. The other video clips are then selected to prepare the parent to successfully manage the vulnerability of learning about his or her particular linchpin issue. The clips often help parents see specific needs of their child in a positive light and know that they have some competency regarding the linchpin problem.

The theory of change at the heart of the COS protocol focuses upon establishing a shift in the parent state of mind ("Shark Music") regarding both the child's attachment needs and how the parent thinks about him- or herself while responding to those needs. Shelly's defensive management of her "Shark Music" led her to "give up" when her son needed her to take charge. Jacob's rejection and anger triggered a visceral sense in her of being a child who feels unloved and unlovable, especially within a context that included separation–autonomous action. To avoid the painful affect, she abdicated her parental authority. For Shelly to take charge she had to rely on her own internal resources and function autonomously without any immediate external support. To do this she needed to be confident that, even though her son is rejecting her in the moment, he still loves and needs her. Sadly, her implicit relational knowing did not support an autonomous sense of self and interfered with her choice.

During the groups, Shelly described a history that indicated that when she acted independently with her mother she was often rejected. Shelly learned that to keep her caregiver available she must diminish autonomy, curtail exploration (top half of Circle), and rely on her mother's thoughts and feelings and not her own. She associated self-assertion with painful feelings of rejection, abandonment, and being left alone because she was bad. Her "Shark Music" included the danger, pain, and negative self-representations experienced when she attempted to claim autonomous functioning. Hence, Shelly experienced this same fear when claiming her parental role of providing guidance for her son.

Shelly's internal working model (Bowlby, 1988) was split into two discrete and unintegrated portraits: when she was dependant and accepted by someone whom she loved she was "good," and when she was on her own or had to stand on her convictions in the face of disapproval she was "bad." Therefore, for Shelly autonomy in the service of a separate self was avoided at all costs. Unbeknownst to her, the cost to her son was the security of his attachment and the cost to her was the loss of a self-directed life.

Given the above analysis of Shelly's internal world and the way it manifests in her relationship with Jacob, the following goals for Shelly's Phase 1 tape review were chosen:

• To help her see that her son needed her at all points on the COS, both top and bottom. He needed her when he was exploring and he needed her when he was upset and distressed. Knowing this was contrary to her belief that Jacob's need for her was provisional and depended upon whether she was "good" (dependent on his approval) or "bad" (standing on her convictions). For Shelly to know that she was indispensable would challenge her internal working model and thus create a state of emotional disequilibrium for her. In contrast, this knowledge had the potential to be experienced as good news because it could disentangle her from the sense that her son's connection with her was conditional.

• To assist Shelly in acknowledging the hurt she felt when Jacob did not include her in his exploration. It was hoped that talking about her pain would set the stage for the more difficult process, in the next tape review, of confronting how she manages her pain and the insecurity it creates for herself and her son.

• To support Shelly in recognizing that there were already moments when she employed a clear, firm voice and acted "bigger, stronger, wiser, and kind." When she claimed her rightful position as Jacob's mother, he followed her lead. To share this moment on tape would directly confront her current, distorted representation of herself as an incompetent adult. It would also be an example of Shelly demonstrating her "underused capacity." This key moment, in which she told her son to "take that out of your mouth," stood in sharp contrast to the way she usually pleaded with him.

Shelly appeared nervous as she began her first tape review. Fortunately, she had seen other parents successfully complete this review process. The group had been supportive during each parent's review and this gave her some confidence. As she prepared to watch her clips, she shared a recent memory of almost coming to tears when Jacob told her he missed her. The other parents in the group reinforced how important she was to her son.

The first set of clips showed rare moments of Jacob successfully using his mother to explore his environment. The clips showed Jacob on the "top half" of the Circle, cueing Shelly for the functions of "help me" and "enjoy with me." Brief clips of positive interactions in which Shelly responded appropriately to Jacob's need were chosen. After each clip, Shelly and the group identified Jacob's need and I[1] pointed out how much Jacob used her as a secure base resource. This section of the review proceeded well with Shelly feeling valued. Given her internal model, being regarded in such a positive light was also somewhat confusing. I talked to Shelly about how much Jacob turned to her as a source of security as he explored his environment. She responded, "I never thought of it that way." For Shelly to know the extent of her worth to Jacob, especially when she was being competent, evoked not only good feelings but also discomfort, from a lifetime belief that she was "not loved and cared for" and therefore unworthy.

Helping parents consider their child's needs in a new light is essential in the COS protocol. So many parents in high-risk populations do not know the extent of their worth to their children. This often stems from parents not feeling valued during their own development. Starting from the belief that they are not of value, parents often project negative attributions onto their child's expression of need ("He doesn't like me" or "She never wants me"). Unexamined, this negative attribution (Fraiberg et al., 1975) organizes their experience of their child's needs all around the COS.

The next clip was selected to explore a more vulnerable process for Shelly. She appeared hurt when Jacob wanted to play without her. She put it this way: "He wants to explore. I want to explore with him but he doesn't want me to explore with him, so I am kind of mad he doesn't want me to." When one of the other parents asked her to talk about the look on her face when her son did not want to play with her, Shelly became mildly defensive and said, "I wanted to play with him . . . OK?" I responded to her painful look with "What comes across is it looks like

---

[1]The treating therapist for this case was Bert Powell, and the treatment section uses first person to describe the process.

you felt hurt." She softened and said, "Yeah." While identifying all the ways Jacob needed her, I explored her feelings of rejection and wondered if she knew just how important she was to him. Shelly softened further and was able to acknowledge that sometimes when he wants to play alone she feels hurt and unimportant to him. Shelly was willing to talk about the vulnerable feeling of rejection associated with her son's exploration and in so doing, demonstrated essential capacities for change.

The COS uses the acronym R-A-R to characterize three essential ingredients of change.

- The first "R" stands for "relationship" and represents the therapist and parent negotiating a safe "holding environment" (Winnicott, 1965) relationship. The therapist and the group become a secure base from which the parent can explore.
- "A" stands for "affect regulation" (Cassidy, 1994). Through the co-regulation of emotion with a caregiver, children learn strategies of both emotional self-regulation and of managing emotions in intimate relationships. Parents bring to the group their own unique history of how emotions are managed. During the group, some aspect of how they manage chronic painful affects will inevitably be challenged. When a parent begins to allow the therapist to be part of a painful experience (feelings and memories associated with their "Shark Music"), a new possibility emerges. Feelings that have chronically interfered with their ability to respond to their child can now be "held" (Winnicott, 1965) by the therapist, the group, and the parent. This experience of shared understanding and co-regulation of difficult emotion lays the foundation for the parent to provide more secure parenting.
- The last "R" stands for "reflection." When a parent engages in reflective dialogue with the therapist while simultaneously feeling the emotions associated with his or her "Shark Music," therapeutic change is furthered.

In summary, change occurs as parents risk being in the "shark-infested waters" of specific, painful, previously unexplored and unregulated attachment feelings. By allowing someone to be in that same water with them, and reflecting on the experience, a therapeutic shift becomes possible.

The final clip reviewed was of the toy cleanup and highlighted a moment in which Shelly directed Jacob to take a toy out of his mouth and Jacob promptly responded. At first, Shelly had trouble seeing her strength. The other mothers in the group saw Shelly's competency and talked about it in a positive manner. After watching the clip again, Shelly finally saw the difference in her demeanor. I gave the name "The Voice" to her firm and commanding tone as she took charge. For Shelly, using "The Voice" became a metaphor for having confidence in herself and knowing her importance as a parent. Showing her a moment in which she took charge revealed that the issue was not whether she had competence, but whether or not she was willing to utilize what she already knew how to do. No matter what parenting skill she learned, if her state of mind was one of hurt, rejection, and lack of importance her son would have a power with her that reduced her to functioning like a hurt child whom he did not have to take seriously.

At the end of this first tape review, Shelly stated that until now she had never thought about how his cues and miscues affected her and she liked learning about it. This is a significant moment in a parent's work. Shelly was seeing procedural information for the first time. Without the videotape, she would likely never have seen or believed the interpretations offered. Procedural information is not readily accessible and video offers a powerful way for parents to see that which they do not see in their daily lives.

Over the next 6 weeks, Shelly attended the group on a regular basis and actively participated in group discussions. In the beginning of each group, the parents were asked to share "Circle stories," which were focused on incidents during the week in which they noticed their child using them as a secure base and a safe haven. Shelly's stories focused on using "The Voice." She was confused because sometimes her voice worked and sometimes it did not. The other members of the group encouraged her to claim her "voice" with her son. As she explored her relationship with Jacob, she fluctuated between feeling strong and helpless.

In week 11, Shelly participated in her second videotape review. The plan was to help Shelly see how she collapsed during moments when her son was angry and needed her to take charge and to help him organize his feelings. The consequences of her collapsing were that her son had to manage his distress alone and she felt small and powerless. Shelly was particularly anxious in the beginning of her review. She had already seen several other parents explore their "Shark Music" and she anticipated being exposed as a "bad" parent.

She began the group by citing a recent example of not knowing how to manage her son when he was angry. I said to her, "For some reason when your son is upset he doesn't know how to use you to calm down . . . what's going on that when he is upset he wants to push you away and you want to help him?" Shelly appeared hurt as she nodded her head in agreement and said, "That is what I do with my mom." Commenting on Shelly's current struggle helped her recognize the parallel between how her son is with her and how she is with her mother. Many of the COS parents begin to recognize this intergenerational connection between how they were raised and how they now raise their children. With her statement, Shelly was expanding her reflective capacity and beginning the process of establishing a "choice point" where there previously had not been a choice. Until the implicit is made explicit and procedural memory is given language, chronic patterns of insecure interaction remain hidden outside the realm of choice.

Shelly continued, "This makes me feel bad—when he wants me to leave, it hurts. I am trying to comfort him, and he is telling me to go away and I don't want you to be here." The other parents were touched by Shelly's struggle and they shared their experience of difficult moments of calming and helping their own children. I focused the discussion on the value of "Time-In Parenting" (Weininger, 1998), which emphasizes providing relationship for children when they are upset. Shelly took the position that she wanted to help Jacob calm, but he would not allow her to do so. Talking about her relationship in this fashion exposed her linchpin issue of allowing Jacob to be in charge of the relationship to avoid her own fear of being abandoned by him. I sensed her anxiety and decided to modify the protocol by giving Shelly the central message of the tape review *before* she watched the tape. Usually parents are eased into knowing their "Shark Music" by watching the chosen video clips for that review. The hope was that once she understood where the session was going, she might be able to calm her fear of being exposed as a bad parent and become more accessible to the learning process. I softly but firmly stated, "I think that when he needs you he gets controlling, and when you allow yourself to be controlled it scares him." Shelly began to cry, closed her eyes, and tried to gain control of her feelings. She did not speak until she had contained her feelings, and only then did she open her eyes and look at me. In the intensity of the moment, Shelly went inward, closing off from the relationship, and thus revealed her procedural memory of not reaching out to others when she is overwhelmed with feeling. Salvador Minuchin, a prominent family therapist, once stated, "History is always present in the moment." Shelly was showing her history of learning to cope with pain alone.

SHELLY: I know he is very controlling and becomes more and more every day.

THERAPIST: That is what I want to help you with.

SHELLY: I know I am supposed to be the one who is in control but I am not. He is the one who controls me . . .

THERAPIST: When he is being this little controlling guy I think he is afraid, and if you can see that you are the person he needs to be bigger, stronger, and kind and he is the scared one, it might help a lot.

Shelly's tears had lessened and the group members explored the idea that behind a child's angry, controlling behavior is fear and the need for a strong caregiver. Shelly's struggle touched all the parents and they talked about their own struggles with their children. When the time came to watch her tape, she indicated that she was ready.

The initial goal for the session was for Shelly to review how important she was to her son. Vignettes were shown in which Jacob was excited in his play with her, and moments when he missed and needed her when she was out of the room. Since Jacob did not show he needed his mom in a direct manner Shelly needed to develop a more sophisticated eye to see his distress. Jacob had learned to miscue his mother when he needed her by acting as if he did not miss or need her for comfort and care. Jacob revealed his distress through subtle changes in the tone and tempo of his play. When his mother was in the room his play was animated and lively, and when she wasn't in the room his play was flat and without focus. Until Shelly recognized Jacob needed her, it was not possible to explore how they negotiated his attachment needs during the reunion. One other clip was employed to emphasize his need. It was the brief moment when he was alone and he turned suddenly and gazed at the one-way mirror with a sad expression on his face. Since the moment was so brief, a bit of creative editing was called for to make that moment have more impact. A single video frame of Jacob's longing face was projected on the television screen as I asked Shelly, "What does this say to you?" Shelly softened and said, "Where is my mom?" She saw his need.

Shelly was now caught in an emotional dilemma as she began to perceive Jacob's needs in a new light. If she accepted her importance, she felt needed and cared for but she was also exposed to the painful knowledge that this positive feeling had been rare and missing for her during much of her life. Even though she saw his need, her knowledge was fragile and after a few minutes, Shelly reframed his need of her as "just" not pushing her away. She saw his need but to protect herself from the pain of her history she restructured her perception so that it was only a momentary lack of rejection.

James Masterson (1993) calls the defensive process of inhibiting positive self-care because it evokes painful memories the "Triad." Risking new, supportive, and more secure perceptions and behaviors, which he terms self-activation, evokes abandonment–depression, which leads to defense. Masterson's abandonment–depression is more than just depression; it is the whole array of emotions associated with profound failures in primary attachment relationships. For Shelly to have a positive image of her relationship with her son when he was not taking care of her required her to autonomously self-activate and step outside her defensive internal working model. When her defensive working model does not protect her, she is vulnerable to historic feelings of abandonment and being unloved. She defended against these feelings by going back to seeing her son in a negative light as the rejecting other, once more reenacting the historic scenario of having been rejected when she self-activated because she was bad. In other words, to protect herself from the historic pain of feeling alone Shelly gave up seeing her son and herself in a positive manner and settled for the familiar experience of feeling connected and small. As parents risk change, tracking the "Triad" is essential to help them solidify their painfully gained knowledge. I gently challenged her limited way of seeing her son and group members joined in, supporting the idea of her value and his need of her. With her fragile insight about her value to Jacob, she was as ready as she was going to be in this session to confront her "Shark Music."

Shelly's linchpin clip was the second reunion in the SSP. Jacob's attachment behaviors were activated before she came into the room. When she returned, he kept his back to her and only responded minimally to her questions. Shelly got on the floor and tried to join him in his play, but when she touched the toys, Jacob told her "No." After several failed attempts to join him, she reenacted her procedural belief system by once again feeling rejected, giving up, and moving back to her chair. Jacob, feeling his unacknowledged need for her, immediately called her back and directed her to a toy. Jacob was showing a controlling pattern of managing his attachment needs by acting both controlling and rejecting.

During her second tape review, when she viewed the videotape of Jacob keeping his back to her when she first entered the room, Shelly was able to say that he was behaving this way because he was hurt. This new depiction of Jacob was a positive sign because it implied that she was holding her image of him as small and hurt instead of her more defensive image of him as big and rejecting. I said, "When he needs you he manages his feelings by becoming rejecting and controlling." Shelly answered, "It's kind of hurtful because I want to play with him. I want to play with him and he doesn't want me to and so "I just give up." In this statement, Shelly disclosed her linchpin problem. When she felt rejected and unwanted, she gave up and this left Jacob without a mother who was available to provide him with care and stability. When Shelly collapsed, it frightened Jacob and he managed his fear by becoming more angry and controlling. His anger frightened Shelly and she collapsed even more. I said, "You are so hurt, and having to deal with your own pain of rejection it makes it hard for you to be bigger, stronger, wiser, and kind . . . he needs you and the last person in the world he wants to get rid of is you, but that is what he acts like. . . . He is saying he missed you, and he doesn't know how to show you his need, so he shows you controlling. After a pause, I asked, "What is it like to think this way?" Shelly responded, "Relief that what he actually needs is me. I am not giving it to him, but in a way, I did not know, but now I do."

Shelly's face revealed both positive feelings and pain as she talked. The session ended with watching the "Voice" clip from the Phase 1 tape review again and reminding Shelly of her competency. Shelly felt threatened by the challenge the clip represented and stated she has tried to have "The Voice" but it doesn't work. I said, "When you are hurt by Jacob's rejection you end up needing acceptance from him and that turns everything around, with him having more power than you. He has power with his rejection and it is a power you can not give him because it will frighten him and it hurts you . . . you are everything to him and you just have to know this." Shelly said, "It is hard" and began to cry.

As she cried, I asked her if there was anything she needed. She covered her face and emotionally withdrew. After a few minutes, I decided to comment on her way of managing her emotions by saying, "I can see that you are used to sorting things out alone and today is an important step because you are sorting this out with us." Group members spontaneously gave her support and offered to be available to Shelly outside of the group when she needed to talk about her feelings.

At the end of the session, Shelly disclosed, "I guess I feel that I did something wrong . . . 'cause I feel it is my fault that I did something wrong to make him feel so angry." Once again, to protect herself from the self-activation involved in using her recent insights, she defended by dropping into the familiar emotional process of thinking of herself as bad. If her defense is successful, her new learning will cease. In the last few minutes of the group I struggled to help Shelly consider that she did nothing wrong, was not to blame, and in fact was supporting herself and doing something right by looking at her relationship with her son. I concluded the group by stating, "The goal for every parent is to take what is good from where we came from and to leave what did not work behind and to do something a little better for their child and that is what you are doing." Shelly ended the group teetering between self-support and self-blame.

To gather new therapeutic material for the third tape review, the parent and child are videotaped a week or two after the parents' second ("Shark Music") tape review. The taping uses a modified SSP that starts with blowing bubbles, has one separation, one reunion, a reading time, and a cleanup. The primary goal of this videotaping is to find moments in which the parents are beginning to manage their "Shark Music" and be more successful with their linchpin issue. The majority of parents show both improvement and continuing struggle. The last review has the overall feeling of celebrating the parents' growth while acknowledging current issues with which they are struggling.

Shelly showed progress in taking charge with Jacob in several episodes of the videotape. When playing with the bubbles, Jacob started frantically popping the bubbles and waving his bubble wand so rambunctiously that Shelly had to set limits. She was able to take charge and help Jacob slow down while maintaining the enjoyment of the play. When Shelly had to take charge and get Jacob to put the toys away, her stance went from a plea of "Can you help me?," proceeded to a modest directive of "Let's pick up the toys," and successfully ended with the take-charge position of "Put that toy away." Shelly was revealing both her new capacity and her struggle. Jacob was much more cooperative with her throughout the videotaping.

When Shelly left Jacob during the separation, he showed distress. When she returned to the room he miscued her by acting like all he needed was help with a toy. With the new insight she had gained she was able to maintain emotionally even responsiveness to him rather than "giving up" when he was frustrated. This is a crucial phase for all the parents. When parents first change their caregiving behavior, the child does not immediately provide them with reinforcement for their efforts. The relationship goes through a transitional phase in which the parent needs to maintain the new caregiving behavior while helping the child learn that the new behavior is reliable. Jacob's change will only consolidate if he knows that his mom is going to claim her rightful position as mother and more often than not support herself as the parent in their relationship. A significant goal of this last tape review is to give the parent support for maintaining the change that has been set in motion.

Shelly appeared less anxious and more available in her Phase 3 tape review. When she reviewed the vignette of her coming back into the room and Jacob miscuing her, she stated that she did not think of him as needing her when she returned. Again, Shelly's "Shark Music" kept her from recognizing her value to her son. I said to her, "I think this is your growing edge . . . to recognize how much he does need you. You underestimate your importance in all these ways and because of that you don't see his need." Shelly agreed and indicated she felt good thinking about how important she was. She revealed that she feels uncomfortable when Jacob tells her he loves her and her discomfort stems from the fact that she has never had this from anyone. She recalled a memory of her uncle's death. She tried to hug her mother at the time of the funeral and her mother pushed her away. Shelly saw that learning to accept Jacob's affection is an essential part of overcoming her "Shark Music." Shelly's struggle emphasized one of the key themes we, as clinicians, have learned from many of the parents involved in COS: *It not only hurts to give that which you did not get, but it also hurts to receive it.* I said to her, "This is your growing area, he is loosening up a little in terms of showing you affection . . . you were worried about that and now that he is doing it you are hearing 'Shark Music.' "

When she first observed the toy cleanup she was unable to see her increased firmness with Jacob. After viewing the tape twice and with the group's support, she barely saw that she was taking charge. Even though Shelly had started to behave differently, she had to struggle to see herself in a new and positive light. Her older representations of herself as little and bad colored her perceptions.

The postintervention SSP occurred 1 week after the program ended. Throughout the procedure, Shelly acted less tentative and more supportive of Jacob's exploration and did not give up when Jacob acted resistant or controlling. Jacob sought contact with his mother during the reunions but miscued her by showing some resistance to her care. Jacob's attachment was scored as Secure (B-4). The preschool scoring manual describes the B-4 category in the following way: "The behavior of children in this group is generally secure, but elements of immature, dependent, ambivalent, or resistant behavior are also present." Jacob had begun to use his mother as a secure base and as a safe haven and showed mild miscuing (resistance) as he did so. In the postintervention SSP, Shelly followed Jacob's exploration and did not intrude in his interests. With Shelly less intrusive, Jacob was less aggressive. Shelly appeared more confident during the reunions and Jacob far less controlling. When he was controlling Shelly maintained her position as the "bigger, stronger, wiser, and kind" parent and Jacob appeared to be merely playing at being controlling. In the first few moments of the second reunion, Jacob maintained sustained eye contact with Shelly as he greeted and talked to her. During the preintervention reunions, Jacob hardly looked at his mother at all. He can now increasingly turn to his mother to help him with his emotions and to support his exploration. His anticipated developmental trajectory with his newfound secure attachment to his mother is substantially more positive than it was when his attachment was insecure-other with signs of controlling and avoidance.

In the postintervention COSI, Shelly demonstrated her understanding that Jacob needed her when she was out of the room. She said, "When he was alone he looked around for me" and that he was "excited to have me come back." She continued, "I knew he wanted and missed me." Shelly saw his need of her and this represented a change in her representations of her son. Shelly struggled more with her own self-representation oscillating between thinking of herself as "good" and "bad." Her relationship with herself is far more entrenched, representing a lifetime of experience. Seeing that Jacob needed her created a crisis in her internal working model. Shelly anticipates rejection and abandonment when she feels worthy of care. Her resolution to the internal conflict of both feeling positive and threatened by her son's need of her is central to lasting change.

In her work on adult attachment Main coined the term "earned secure." This refers to adults who were raised in obvious adversity but had the resilience to develop a secure state of mind as an adult. The key to earned security is having self-reflection, which enables adults to coherently organize a perspective regarding their developmental history, and the capacity to acknowledge the impact past experiences have on current relationships. The more Shelly shares her struggle with trusted adults and finds perspective regarding her painful history, the more she will continue on the road to "earned security." This is, of course, where ongoing therapeutic support would be of value to her.

When asked what gives her the most difficulty in her relationship with Jacob she cited exactly the same issue as in her initial COSI, discipline, and told the same story of Jacob once more demanding ice cream for breakfast. This time she said, "You've got to learn someday you can't have ice cream for breakfast . . . then we switched to eggs." When asked how she thought Jacob was thinking about her in this incident she replied, "He didn't like me because I didn't let him have what he wants." When asked how she thought about herself in this incident she replied, "Good, I guess, I didn't give in and let him have the ice cream." When describing this conflict in the initial COSI she feared her son would hate her if she took charge. To be able to hold any positive image of herself as she appropriately takes charge, especially in the face of her son's rejection, is crucial progress.

At the end of the interview, she was asked how participation in the project had affected her relationship with her son. She stated with positive emotion, "He cues [me] when he needs something like a hug when I come into the room . . . when I pick him up from day care he is excited to see me and he never used to do that before . . . he is all happy to see me!" For her son to show her his need so openly, when previously he did not, indicates that Shelly is accepting and welcoming of his affection.

CLOSING REMARKS AND CONCLUSION

Shelly and Jacob's story represents a significant category of parents who are in need of early intervention. To understand Shelly's process is to understand the separation-sensitive caregiver who maintains a role-reversed relationship with his or her child out of fear. This parent needs emotional support from the child to feel stable, suffers emotional dysregulation when called upon to take a stance that requires autonomous functioning, and thus avoids taking charge. In such a role-reversed relationship, the child is compelled to organize the relationship, which is often done in an angry and controlling manner. Such a child needs to feel safe but often evokes from adults punitive discipline that only reinforces the problem.

In the COSI and during the protocol Shelly described her relationship with her mother as anxious and rejecting. To cope, she learned to attend to her mother's needs and not to her own. If she developed her own interests as an autonomous person, her mother would be angry and even less available. Shelly became hypervigilant for any experience that might lead to her feeling abandoned and organized her life in very specific ways to avoid self-assertion. For her, self-assertion implied inevitable rejection. In the mind of a young child learning the procedure of relationship, her rather primitive logic went something like this: "My mom rejects me each time I do something on my own. This must mean that I am bad when I act on my own behalf." Thus, she developed an internal working model that was organized around her fear of separation-as-rejection. For her to feel separated from someone who loved her meant that she was alone, helpless, and without internal resources. It is no surprise that when she was an adolescent, she was so depressed that she fantasized about dying as a way to end her pain. As a teenager, she was vulnerable to any boy who acted remotely as if he liked her and was easy to manipulate with threats of abandonment. Fortunately she experienced the birth of her son at age 16 as a wake-up call to make a life for herself and him. Unfortunately, she did not know what to do and turned to him to take care of her in ways that interfered with his security.

Shelly's therapy is also quintessential for role-reversed separation-sensitive parents. Her first challenge was to see her son's behavior as an expression of his needs. Her "empathic shift" (Cooper, Hoffman, Powell, & Marvin, 2005) was to see Jacob's angry and controlling behavior as a sign that he needed her. The next challenge was for her to see the manner in which she gave up on Jacob as a way to protect herself from feeling alone and bad. The therapeutic message was that she had the wherewithal to take charge and manage her procedural fear associated with having an autonomous self. Shelly was much stronger than she believed and discovered that she had a "Voice" that not only opened a door with her son but also formed positive relationships with friends and ultimately helped her negotiate a different relationship with her mother.

Approximately 1 year after the intervention, a newspaper reporter who was doing a story on the COS interviewed Shelly's group. During the interview, Shelly was far more animated, confidant, and vocal than she had been a year prior. The mothers were affectionate with each other during the interview and Shelly accepted their positive statements about the gains she had made, both with her son and with her mother.

SHELLY: At first I was quiet, I was more afraid than anything but then . . . I blossomed.

REPORTER: What were you afraid of?

SHELLY: Opening up my life to people that I did not know.

REPORTER: What about the program let you do that?

SHELLY: Support, the people, and the feedback from everybody.

REPORTER: Anything in particular you learned from the program that you would like to share?

SHELLY: What helped me the most was my voice. Knowing that mom voice, that sternly says no you can't do this and sticking with it. . . . He was putting a toy into his mouth and I said get it out and he automatically just dropped it and put it away. I never knew that.

When Shelly said she blossomed she did so with a somewhat shy but positive demeanor. For her to speak in such a positive way concerning her identity in a group setting with a reporter present represented a change in how she thought about herself. By recognizing and accepting her value to her son and developing her strength, she had begun to discover a sense of her own innate worth. During this interview, Shelly recalled the exact (linchpin) moment of change for her in discovering that she had the strength to take charge with her son, thus providing him the security he needed. She came across as a young woman who is in the process of finding her voice, learning she has something to say and that others are interested in her opinions.

The COS program was the initial part of the change process. She continued in Head Start for 1 year after the program ended with a talented teacher and a family service coordinator, both of whom supported her changes on a daily basis. Most of the parents from the COS group also remained at the site for the year following the program and became a support network for one another. The initial change process that began in the group was shaped and reinforced over the following year by COS-trained staff and parents. We believe that in order for changes to endure parents need to be involved in a support network that knows and appreciates a relationship- and attachment-oriented approach to parenting.

The Minnesota Longitudinal Study (Sroufe et al., 2005) found that having an emotionally supportive relationship with an adult partner was a significant protective factor in not passing on abuse and neglect to the next generation. If Shelly selects a partner who is supportive, the changes she developed in the program will likely solidify into long-term patterns. If she partners with an unsupportive, hostile partner, her changes will most likely not endure. Young single mothers with insecure/disorganized backgrounds need help and support in making one of the most important decisions in their lives, choosing a supportive partner. Their insecure history predicts that without ongoing support they may well select unsupportive mates. The particular COS program Shelly went through only minimally addressed this issue. Work is now being explored within the context of newer approaches in the COS protocol to develop learning modules designed to address this crucial issue. If Shelly can hold on to her reflective capacity, remember her value, and maintain the supportive network she currently has, she has a good chance of staying on her path of giving Jacob that which she did not receive. We want to thank Shelly for her commitment, her vulnerability, and her courage to confront her fear.

REFERENCES

Aber, J. L., Slade, A., Cohen, L., & Meyer, J. (1989, April). *Parental representations of their toddlers: Their relationship to parental history and sensitivity and toddler security.* Paper presented at the biennial meeting of the Society for Research in Child Development, Kansas City, MO.

Ainsworth, M. D. S., Blehar, M. C., Waters, E., & Wall, S. (1978). *Patterns of attachment: Psychological study of the Strange Situation.* Hillsdale, NJ: Erlbaum.

Bollas, C. (1987). *The shadow of the object.* New York: Columbia University Press.

Bowlby, J. (1988). *A secure base: Clinical applications of attachment theory.* London: Routledge.

Cassidy, J. (1994). Emotion regulation: Influences of attachment relationships. In N. Fox (Ed.), The development of emotion regulation. *Monographs of the Society for Research in Child Development, 59*(2–3, Serial No. 240), 228–249.

Cassidy, J., & Marvin, R. S. (1992). *A system for classifying individual differences in the attachment behavior of 2½- to 4½-year-old children.* Unpublished coding manual, University of Virginia, Charlottesville.

Cooper, G., Hoffman, K., Marvin, R., & Powell, B. (1997). *The Circle of Security Interview.* Unpublished materials, Marycliff Institute, Spokane, WA.

Cooper, G., Hoffman, K., & Powell, B. (1998). *Caregiver core sensitivities* [Handout]. Marycliff Institute, Spokane, WA.

Cooper, G., Hoffman, K., Powell, B., & Marvin, R. (2005). The Circle of Security intervention: Differential diagnosis and differential treatment. In L. J. Berlin, Y. Ziv, L. M. Amaya-Jackson, & M. T. Greenberg (Eds.), *Enhancing early attachments: Theory, research, intervention, and policy* (pp. 127–151). New York: Guilford Press.

Fonagy, P., Steele, H., & Steele, M. (1991). Maternal representations of attachment during pregnancy predict the organization of infant–mother attachment at one year of age. *Child Development, 62,* 891–905.

Fonagy, P., Steele, M., Steele, H., Higgitt, A., & Target, M. (1994). The theory and practice of resilience. *Journal of Child Psychology and Psychiatry and Allied Disciplines, 35,* 231–257.

Fonagy, P., Steele, M., Steele, H., & Target, M. (1997). *Reflective-functioning manual, Version 4.1, for application to Adult Attachment Interviews.* Unpublished coding manual, University of London.

Fraiberg, S. H., Adelson, E., & Shapiro, V. (1975). Ghosts in the nursery: A psychoanalytic approach to the problem of impaired mother–infant relationships. *Journal of the American Academy of Child Psychiatry, 14,* 387–422.

George, C., Kaplan, N., & Main, M. (1985). *The Adult Attachment Interview.* Unpublished manuscript, University of California, Berkeley.

Hoffman, K., Cooper, G., Marvin, R., & Powell, B. (1997). *Seeing with Joey.* Unpublished manuscript, Marycliff Institute, Spokane, WA.

Hoffman, K., Marvin, R., Cooper, G., & Powell, B. (2006) Changing toddlers' and preschoolers' attachment classifications: The Circle of Security intervention. *Journal of Consulting and Clinical Psychology, 74*(6), 1017–1026.

Kernberg, O. F. (1975). *Borderline conditions and pathological narcissism.* New York: Jason Aronson.

Kohut, H. (1971). *The analysis of the self.* New York: International Universities Press.

Liotti, G. (1992). Disorganized/disoriented attachment in etiology of dissociative disorders. *Dissociation, 5,* 196–204.

Lyons-Ruth, K. (1998). Implicit relational knowing: Its role in development and psychoanalytic treatment. *Infant Mental Health Journal, 19,* 282–289.

Main, M., & Hesse, E. (1990). Parents' unresolved traumatic experiences are related to infant disorganized attachment status: Is frightened and/or frightening parental behavior the linking mechanism? In M. T. Greenberg, D. Cicchetti, & E. M. Cummings (Eds.), *Attachment in the preschool years: Theory, research, and intervention* (pp. 161–182). Chicago: University of Chicago Press.

Marvin, R., Cooper, G., Hoffman, K., & Powell, B. (2002). The Circle of Security project: Attachment-based intervention with caregiver–preschool child dyads. *Attachment and Human Development, 1*(4), 107–124.

Masterson, J. (1976). *The psychotherapy of the borderline adult.* New York: Brunner/Mazel.

Masterson, J. (1993). *The emerging self.* New York: Brunner/Mazel.

Masterson, J., & Klein, R. (Eds.). (1995). *The disorders of the self: New therapeutic horizons, the Masterson approach.* New York: Brunner/Mazel.

Sroufe, L. A., Egeland, B., Carlson, E. A., & Collins, W. A. (2005). *The develop-

ment of the person: The Minnesota Study of Risk and Adaptation from Birth to Adulthood. New York: Guilford Press.

van IJzendoorn, M. H., Schuengel, C., & Bakermans-Kranenburg, M. J. (1999). Disorganized attachment in early childhood: Meta-analysis of precursors, concomitants, and sequelae. *Development and Psychopathology, 11,* 225–249.

Weininger, O. (1998). *Time-in parenting strategies.* New York: ESF.

Winnicott, D. W. (1965). *The maturational processes and the facilitating environment.* London: Hogarth Press.

CHAPTER EIGHT

Challenging Children's Negative Internal Working Models

Utilizing Attachment-Based Treatment Strategies in a Therapeutic Preschool

DOUGLAS F. GOLDSMITH

Children who are identified as insecurely attached to their primary caregiver tend to develop relationships with adults and peers that are characterized by mistrust, anger, and anxiety. Over time, these negative representations begin to color all of their relationships, causing these children to respond to even minimal provocation with reactive aggression, or conversely to rely on defensive withdrawal in order to modulate their emotional needs. This chapter will describe how parent–child psychotherapy is used in tandem with a therapeutic preschool program that incorporates attachment-based treatment strategies to challenge children's negative internal working models of relationships. Parent–child psychotherapy sessions address negative parental representations of the child and focus on helping parents develop the emotional sensitivity, communication skills, and structure within the home environment that will foster a secure relationship. The child, simultaneously, attends the therapeutic preschool where nurturing interactions with adults are used to challenge the children's view of adults as punitive and unavailable, and through these interactions the children learn that adults can be utilized to solve problems, calm their affective storms, and support the development of positive interactions with peers.

Bowlby (1982) theorized that during the second and third years of life, as children are beginning to explore their environment in circles that extend beyond their primary caregiver, they construct internal working models that will help them predict how their primary caregiver as well as significant others in their environment can be expected to behave. Built upon their experiences with caregivers, internal working models guide children as they evaluate interpersonal situations and develop plans for how to respond and behave in new environments and relationships. In essence, relationship experiences during their first few years of life create a roadmap that children utilize as they navigate new relationships and environments. Children who have enjoyed sensitive and responsive caregivers are able to explore their environments confidently and are willing to seek help when necessary, having learned that their caregivers are readily available to help soothe them and repair any emotional disruptions. In contrast, children who have not experienced available and reliable caregiving learn to perceive the environment as unreliable and, as a result, fear exploration or, conversely, engage others with aggression and negativity (Bretherton, 2005).

Bowlby (1988) believed that children's dysfunctional interactions with others in environments such as preschool can be explained by recognizing that as children develop they attempt to impose their internal working models on new relationships and across new contexts. Consider, for example, Ricky, a 4-year-old child who is playing calmly with his toy train in the preschool classroom. As another child approaches, Ricky looks up defensively, his brow furrowed and his jaw tightened. These are the external manifestations of his internal working model that has taught him to anticipate hostile interactions rather than friendly approaches to play. He yells at the child to leave him alone while simultaneously jumping up ready to strike. Within seconds the two boys are engaged in an aggressive battle. His therapist rushes over to stop the fight but as she approaches, Ricky turns and begins to spit at her. When she attempts to take his hand to help calm him, he falls to the floor flailing his arms and kicking ferociously. While some may consider Ricky to manifest clear symptoms of an oppositional defiant disorder, a careful review of his early history finds that his mother has struggled with depression since his birth, his parents divorced during his first year, and Ricky has experienced little consistency from his caregivers during his first years of life. Ricky's experience, reflected in his internal working model, has essentially taught him to expect that he is not worthy of loving care from others. In fact, it has created an internalized expectation that interactions with both peers and adults result in angry, unsatisfying, and even hurtful exchanges. As a result, he defensively strikes at his playmate as well as his therapist. He expects that the interaction will fail to provide him with comfort or satisfaction, and preemptively attacks in order to ward off the punitive interaction that he has grown to expect. Understanding that Ricky is an insecurely attached little boy who has developed negative internal working models of his relationships with peers and adults leads to interventions aimed at restoring a positive internal working model of self and others rather than simply extinguishing his aggression.

The need for clinicians to be particularly sensitive to the impact of insecure attachment as a primary issue underlying behavioral and emotional problems in early childhood settings is supported by research. For example, 80–84% of preschool-age children in mental health clinics have been classified as insecure (Greenberg, Spelz, DeKlyen, & Endriga, 1991). In addition, Sroufe (2005) has shown that securely attached children are readily identified by their ability to engage their teachers and peers with positive affect, empathize with others when they are distressed, and sustain cooperative play with their classmates. They enter the early child care environment equipped to master developmental challenges that include learning to play cooperatively with peers, regulating emotions, and responding empathically to peers and adults. Insecurely attached preschoolers, on the other hand, are ill equipped to master these challenges. They tend to exhibit angry outbursts in the preschool classroom and, not surprisingly, show lower sociability and poorer peer relations (Carlson & Sroufe, 1995). They resort to aggressive behavior to modulate interactions and rely heavily on teachers to guide them as they attempt to negotiate play interactions (Sroufe, 2005).

While insecure attachment and subsequent relationship disturbances are best treated through parent–child psychotherapy (Lieberman, 2004; Sameroff, 2004), focusing treatment interventions exclusively on the child's familial relationships fails to take into account the impact of the extension of the child's relational disturbances to adults and peers in the preschool environment. This chapter demonstrates the importance of using a therapeutic preschool program along with parent–child therapy to address the impact of relational disturbances on the child's functioning within the home as well as the preschool environment. In this program the group intervention is utilized to challenge children's attachment strategies and their negative internal working models. The intervention also supports children as they learn to regulate their emotions by learning to verbalize their feelings so that others will better understand, and thus be able to respond to, their wants and needs. The chapter begins with a review of pertinent attachment concepts used in the assessment and formulation of treatment planning and intervention. A case history is then presented in order to highlight attachment interventions in clinical practice.

DEVELOPING A SECURE BASE

Attachment theory focuses on the critical need for infants to develop a secure attachment to their primary caregiver and describes the behaviors necessary, within the context of the relationship, to facilitate a sense of security (Fonagy, 2001). Fostered by emotionally attuned and available caregivers, securely attached infants seek proximity to the attachment figure when confronted with a situation that is frightening, threatening, or anxiety producing. Infants quickly learn that proximity with the caregiver reliably produces a sense of comfort, security, and soothing (Bowlby, 1988). After being soothed, secure infants can resume exploration of their environment unencumbered by distress. This cycle of exploration followed by a return to the caregiver for support occurs with high frequency for infants and toddlers, but becomes less frequent as the child approaches the preschool years. By this age, the urgency for proximity on the part of the child has typically decreased (Bowlby, 1982). Seeking proximity to the caregiver creates feelings of emotional intimacy for the child and the parent. For the child this intimacy enhances the experience of being warmly embraced, and creates the comfort of knowing what it is like to feel understood and supported in a loving relationship. For the caregiver such interactions engender joy from being needed and satisfaction at being able to provide comfort to the child. It is this intimate interaction that differentiates the parent–child relationship from the child's relationship with other caregivers.

Unfortunately, children with insecure attachments resist seeking proximity, and as a result they engage in fewer intimate interactions with their caregiver. As a result, the parent–child dyad begins to feel emotionally distant, evoking parental frustration and anger toward the child. In turn the preschooler ends up feeling isolated and helpless when confronting frightening and frustrating experiences. A negative cycle is quickly perpetuated. If the child stops seeking help and reassurance when anxious or upset, the parent no longer feels needed and appreciated by the child. The ensuing stress for the parent is often projected negatively on the child, as the parent seeks an explanation for the child's lack of intimate outreach. In the clinical setting this projection involves anger toward the child or an admission of not being able to feel close to the child. One mother expressed her frustration, sense of rejection, and unhappiness by saying, "If he was an animal he'd be at the pound by now."

Seeking proximity to the attachment figure is not only necessary for comfort, but plays an important role in the development of emotion regulation from infancy onward. Securely attached children appreciate that their caregiver will be emotionally available and sensitively respond to their needs and signals when they are emotionally aroused. The emotionally attuned caregiver effectively teaches the child that emotional arousal is not necessarily disorganizing and, in the event that the child does feel overwhelmed, restabilization is achieved by seeking proximity to their caregiver (Sroufe, 1995). As a result, securely attached children verbally express their negative affects, expecting that by signaling their emotional distress they will be comforted and reassured by their caregivers (Cicchetti, Ganiban, & Barnett, 1991). The repeated experience of being effectively soothed results in their ability to modulate their emotional state and, consequently, they tend to spend more time engaging in positive exchanges (Cicchetti, Ganiban, & Barnett, 1991). In contrast, children who have not experienced routine comfort tend to be overwhelmed by negative affect, are typically characterized as being angry and hostile in their interactions, and have difficulty directly expressing negative affect (Cassidy & Koback, 1988). Thus, the insecure preschooler exhibits high levels of reactive aggression, which may reflect feelings of anger, but the aggression may also be a reflection of the child's internalized feelings of fear and anxiety. Children placed in "time-out" behind a closed door can become so overwhelmed with feelings of anxiety that, rather than cry and openly express their terror, they become violent and destructive.

The inability to effectively modulate emotion has a negative impact on the primary developmental tasks for preschoolers: learning to engage effectively with peers, manage impulses, and function in a group setting

(Waters & Sroufe, 1983). The secure preschool-age child will freely explore the classroom and willingly turn to adults for support when challenges occur. Children with insecure attachments, however, are less likely to turn to adults, choosing instead to withdraw from conflict or respond with aggression when they feel threatened (Bretherton, 2005). Their experience of caregivers as unresponsive to their inner turmoil (Steele & Steele, 2005) or as being ineffective in calming their affective storms and restoring their emotional equilibrium is projected onto the preschool teacher. The insecure child assumes that the teacher will be equally ineffective. The subsequent resistance to seeking out support creates tension for the preschool teacher, who is constantly distracted by the need to help regulate the child's emotional outbursts and disturbed peer relations. The child's internal working model of adults as ineffective and unavailable therefore has to become a focal point for attachment-based intervention. When considering such working models it is important to examine not only the child's experiences with the caregiver, but also the way the caregiver experiences and views the child. This issue is discussed next.

PARENTAL REPRESENTATIONS OF THE CHILD

The child's internal working model is strongly influenced by the way the parent perceives the child. According to Bowlby (1988), "whatever she [the mother] fails to recognize in him [the child] he is likely to fail to recognize in himself" (p. 132). Of even greater concern to Bowlby (1988) is the risk that the child will respond to negative parental projections. Thus, the parent who experiences the preschool-age child as exhausting and providing little emotional reward may begin to attribute to the child negative characteristics of other family members in an attempt to explain or understand the child's behavior. For example, the child's aggressive behavior will be interpreted as evidence that the child has inherited his father's volatile temper. Likewise, a mother who is infuriated by the frequent power struggles perpetuated by her ex-husband becomes even more inflamed when her 4-year-old son challenges her authority and refuses to respond to her requests. The clinician who fails to appreciate the role of parents' negative representations of their children may prescribe behavioral interventions designed to eradicate children's aggressive or defiant behavior but by doing so may inadvertently provide punitive measures to an already angry and fearful parent. In contrast, understanding parents' negative representations opens the way for the clinician to assist the parent with revising and developing a more accurate and positive working model of the child (see Koren-Karie, Oppenheim, & Goldsmith, Chapter 2, this volume).

The child's psychiatric issues may also compound the negative parental representation of the child. By the time parents seek clinical services for their child they are often exasperated by the confluence of their negative representation and what may be a lack of understanding of the child's actual psychiatric problems. For example, a child with undiagnosed attention problems can be perceived as purposely ignoring parental requests. The child's impulsive anger fuels the parents' negative representation of the child as disrespectful and hostile. The parents, in turn, feel underappreciated and disrespected by the child. As a result, the child who makes a benign request for more time before cleaning up his toys is responded to with impatience and unduly harsh punishment.

The added value of an attachment perspective allows clinicians to evaluate and create attachment-based treatment strategies to effectively address the behavioral problems exhibited by young children in early childhood settings as well as their home environment. The chapter next explores how clinicians utilizing the concepts of secure base behavior and the child's and parent's internal working models are able to effectively treat children's relationship disturbances with parents, siblings, teachers, and peers in the context of a therapeutic preschool program.

RELATIONSHIP-BASED TREATMENT
IN A THERAPEUTIC PRESCHOOL

The Children's Center is a private, not-for-profit mental health center in Salt Lake City, Utah, that utilizes a therapeutic preschool program to teach children to learn to trust adult caregivers to respond to their emotional and developmental needs. The agency provides treatment for families with infants, toddlers, and preschoolers who are struggling with a range of emotional and behavioral problems. Children are referred from preschools, early childhood programs, pediatricians, and governmental services including the Division of Child and Family Services. Diagnostically the children exhibit a wide spectrum of childhood psychiatric diagnoses. The majority of the children have at least an average IQ: those with developmental delays are referred to other clinics. Over two-thirds of the families utilize Medicaid to cover the costs of treatment. The children exhibit high levels of risk factors: 40% have been physically or sexually abused or neglected, 30% have been expelled from preschool or threatened with expulsion, 70% reside with a single parent, and 60% of the parents have a psychiatric diagnosis.

Following a comprehensive developmental history and psychological evaluation, the children are admitted to an intensive therapeutic preschool program that provides treatment for 3 hours, 5 days per week. Over 300 children attend the program annually for treatment that typically lasts for 9 months, though the actual length of treatment is tailored to meet the individual needs of the child. The therapy groups contain nine children and are run by two paraprofessional child therapists who are trained on-site and receive weekly supervision from a licensed clinician. Parents are expected to attend family therapy or parent–child psychotherapy a minimum of twice monthly to help them acquire the capacity to be emotionally available to the child, increase emotional attunement to the child's needs, and ultimately gain the skills to help the child regulate his or her emotions.

The therapeutic preschool program provides a sense of safety and security for the child by serving as a holding environment (Winnicott, 1965) while parents are gaining the skills to provide a secure base at home. A holding environment is deemed essential for children to learn that adults are capable of containing their negative affect while providing an environment that neither stifles nor overwhelms the child's development. The experience of feeling "contained" is critical in order to develop the foundation for challenging the child's negative internal working model of adults as incapable of effectively empathizing with, and responding to, their dysregulated affect.

Children entering the therapeutic preschool program have often been expelled from one or two early childhood programs prior to being referred to the therapeutic preschool. Consequently, they engage in the new relationships with the child therapists prepared for a negative approach, and will often engage in provocative behaviors to immediately test their model of adults as punitive and rejecting. In order to begin to challenge the children's negative internal working model of relationships the staff relies on information from the child's evaluation as well as observations of the child's behavior during the first few days. Using this information they try to demonstrate to the child that they are capable of anticipating and effectively responding to his or her emotional and physical needs.

The foundation of a secure relationship is based on adult interactions that are characterized by understanding and empathically responding to the child's needs. Therefore, establishing a trusting relationship becomes a primary focus from the moment the child enters the group. For example, on the first day of treatment Rachel was accompanied by her mother to the group room. Upon her arrival, the staff member kneeled down to greet her at eye level, smiled, and enthusiastically said, "Hi, Rachel! I'm so glad you're here!" Rachel responded by clinging to her mother and anxiously began whimpering. A new level of understanding was demonstrated to her when the therapist reflected, in a soft tone, "Oh, Rachel, this is a little scary for you but you're going to be OK. Let's have Mommy stay with us for a little bit until you're feeling safe. Maybe you and your mommy could work on a puzzle together at the table." In this brief exchange the child has learned that the therapist is able to accept her anxiety and, as well, is able to effectively read and respond to her nonverbal cues. By using a soft tone and maintaining a respectful physical distance the therapist displayed a level of understanding and sensitivity that is appreciated by the child who has learned to anticipate abrupt, harsh interactions with adults.

To begin to develop trust, the adults must behaviorally challenge the children's working model of them as being unavailable, ineffective, and lacking empathic regard. Nurturing interactions form the basis of secure relationships; but the term "nurturing" is often ambiguous and, as such, is difficult to translate to action. In order to understand how to begin to effectively nurture children the staff is encouraged to consider the concept of an "ideal grandmother" as a guide to assist them in their interactions with the children.

An "ideal grandmother" is imagined to provide unconditional love and acceptance and knows the child so well that she is capable of anticipating the child's needs without the child even needing to verbalize his or her desires. For example, the child's favorite cookies are waiting on the table upon arrival for a visit, because the grandmother *anticipates* that the child will be hungry. She places a warm blanket over a child who is napping, *anticipating* that the child might get cold. By anticipating a child's basic needs the grandmother conveys her ability to effectively understand the child and, even more important, demonstrates that she has been thinking about the child even in the child's absence. The "ideal grandmother" offers a level of understanding and empathic regard that the child experiences as a constant emotional embrace. Such experiences create, for the child, what Pawl (1995) describes as the experience of being held in one's mind. The comfort and delight of being held in mind provide a critical human connection that produces a sense of safety and containment for the child. Such an experience is a critical building block that leads to the development of a secure base for the preschool-age child. For insecurely attached children the attainment of such an experience is an essential step toward fostering the feeling that they are worthy of care and, consequently, begins to challenge previous models that suggest otherwise.

Using this concept as a guide, the staff looks for opportunities to convey a sense of support, safety, and caring within the preschool environment. During the first few months of treatment the staff will offer high levels of support to demonstrate that adults can be turned to for assistance. As trust develops the staff will encourage the children to function more independently in order to help them explore their environment. This sequence is important because developing the basis of adult support is necessary in order for the child to build the confidence to explore the environment independently and "check in" for help when needed. For example, consider the child who at lunchtime is struggling to open his thermos and is increasingly becoming frustrated. The adult reflects, "You're thirsty but you can't get that open. I want to help you so that you can have a drink." This brief interaction will become, in the child's mind, an important step toward seeing him- or herself as valued and adults as capable of providing nurturing and care. Later in treatment, the same behavior will elicit, "It looks like you're having trouble getting that open! You could ask me for help." Toward the end of treatment the therapist will say, "If you need help you know what to do!" Each statement progressively moves the child toward more independent functioning.

Similarly, the staff may offer to help the children with self-care issues such as putting on coats and cleaning up small messes. Putting on a coat can be terribly frustrating for the young child and the children struggle to regulate their emotions, often resulting in an overwhelmed response. The adult might hurry over to the child and exclaim, "Let me help you with that coat. That looks so frustrating for you and I don't want you to be cold outside." Likewise, many children have learned to expect harsh, angry responses when they have accidental spills or messes, and expect a punitive response from the preschool staff as well. Violating the child's expectations, the therapist will instead say, "I will help you clean that up. Spills happen sometimes." By emphasizing the words "I will help" this brief encounter is viewed as an opportunity to challenge the child's model of adults as unhelpful and uncaring. Finally, staff may hurry over to the child who is physically hurt but reluctant to seek assistance and, while soothing the child, point out, "When you fall down and get hurt it scares and upsets you. I'll hold you so I can help you feel better." Children with negative internal working models find these comments to be quite extraordinary. In their experience adults do not have the capacity to help, soothe, and provide patient assistance and support when they are upset and try to regulate their emotions. In fact, it is through these soothing interactions that children learn to incorporate the ability to self-soothe.

Relying on the concepts of emotional mirroring, reflection, and unconditional positive regard the child therapists begin to challenge the child's internal working model of adults as hostile and emotionally unavailable. The children's sense of importance within the context of a relationship is developed when the staff verbalizes that they think about a child even in the child's absence. For example, they may say, "I remembered how much you enjoyed this toy yesterday so I got it out for you this morning." Likewise, staff might reflect, "I was thinking about your long ride to school and thought you might be hungry when you got here so I found some of your favorite cookies." To be thought about in one's absence is viewed by young couples falling in love as the signal that the relationship has assumed a wonderful level of importance in the mind of the other. For the insecurely attached child, it opens up a new realm of feelings regarding the potential for relationships to provide comfort.

During the first weeks and months of treatment the children tend to maintain close physical proximity to the adults because they lack the confidence to explore toys and activities on their own, and also because of their anxiety that exploration might result in harm. As they learn to develop trust in the adults, they begin to explore the environment in increasingly widening circles. By providing high levels of supervision, the staff provides a sense of safety and focus on helping the children explore. The small staff–child ratio of 1:4 is needed in order for them to respond quickly to aggressive outbursts between the children, and respond to aggression by calmly helping the children verbalize their needs. For example, the therapist sees Charlie angrily strike Justin, who is riding on a tricycle. She hurries over and physically holds Charlie back while saying, "You're mad because Justin has the bike. You need to ask for a turn instead of hitting." She then helps Charlie verbalize the desire for a turn and facilitates the sharing of the tricycle to help the boys feel safe, as well as experience the value of the use of verbal skills to get needs met.

This process ultimately helps the insecure child risk venturing away from the adults to explore the environment knowing that help will be provided if necessary. Even more important, the children learn to understand that the adults can effectively be in control of the group, and this challenges their internal working model of adults as being overwhelmed and unavailable.

Exploration for the preschooler also includes the acquisition of preacademic skills, exposure to the inherent joy of learning a new skill, and learning to navigate the world of play and friendships. Through the incorporation of a structured preschool curriculum children are exposed to the academic foundation essential for success in regular early childhood settings and simultaneously acquire a positive sense of self as capable and adept at learning a new skill. Activities are selected that are likely to be met with success in order to minimize frustration and to help develop the child's sense of self as capable and competent (Plenk, 1993).

In the next section I elaborate further on the application of attachment concepts in the therapeutic preschool by presenting the assessment and treatment of a child who had a history of multiple caregiving and trauma prior to being adopted. The adoptive parent sought help because of extreme frustration with her child's aggression at home. Additionally, her child's inability to regulate her emotions was proving to be considerably disruptive for the entire family system, as all of the family members felt like they had to "walk on eggshells" to prevent the child from raging out of control.

THE INITIAL INTERVIEW
AND CASE FORMULATION

The initial clinical interview provides an opportunity to begin to establish the therapeutic relationship, and thus the parents are encouraged to begin to tell their story and share their concerns about the child's behavior and emotional struggles (Hirshberg, 1996). Parents arrive at the interview prepared to discuss their concerns about their child's behavior but are typically uncertain about whether to share information about their own emotional pain. Their personal feelings range from worry and concern about the child's emotional problems to fears that a serious psychiatric disorder will be diagnosed. Additionally, there is trepidation that they might be told nothing is actually wrong with their child, confirming their fear that poor parenting accounts for the child's problems.

They may also worry about exposing their intense pain and anguish over their growing resentment of the child for his or her negative impact on family life.

Keeping these issues in mind, the clinician begins the interview with an invitation to the parents to talk about the concerns that brought them to the clinic. Amy (not her real name) was 2 years old when her adoptive mother brought her to the Children's Center. The information prior to the appointment indicated that she was seeking help due to concerns with Amy's high levels of aggression, constant conflict with the mother's two biological children, and extreme levels of temper outbursts. The following narrative summarizes the initial clinical consultation:

> Amy was screaming and flailing her arms and legs, struggling to get out of her mother's arms as she was carried into the office. Her adoptive mother looked fatigued and was clearly frustrated by Amy's tantrum. After putting her daughter down, she seated herself across from the clinician and exclaimed, "Well, you're getting to see her in her full glory today." Amy was not consoled by being out of her mother's arms and continued to scream and flail on the floor. Glancing briefly toward the clinician, Amy stood up and started to hit her mother on the leg before quickly leaning over and biting her. Her mother screeched and, grabbing Amy by the arms, said, "I can barely stand it anymore!" Her eyes filled with tears as she described daily bouts of tantrums and aggression toward herself, her husband, and her two boys. As she spoke, Amy sat rigidly on her mother's lap and started drinking from her bottle, carefully avoiding eye contact with the therapist. Her face was tense, her brow furrowed, and her posture conveyed tremendous tension coupled with a lack of trust in this novel environment.

It is not unusual for parents to display high levels of emotion early in the assessment process. This can be unsettling for child therapists who believe they must focus the assessment on the child. However, during the initial interview, the clinician must not only be able to engage the child but must also focus on the parent and the parent–child relationship as well. In essence, the parent must feel understood and comforted and given reassurance that help is available. The child, as well, needs to feel understood and experience sufficient empathy that a return to the clinic for more appointments is viewed with positive anticipation.

Amy had clearly shown signs of tremendous discomfort with interpersonal contact, but as she began to relax the clinician attempted to engage Amy in an attempt to increase her comfort. In order to do so, the clinician initiated eye contact and made soothing verbalizations directed toward Amy, who, in response, furrowed her brow and swatted angrily at the air with her clenched fists. She glared at him briefly before averting her eyes and burying her face into her mother's chest. After several minutes, she looked back at the clinician and, when they made eye contact, she again swatted angrily at the air and looked away.

It was clear that Amy was unable, or unwilling, to tolerate any contact. In order for her to begin to develop trust, it was critical to respect her signal to be left alone. Consequently, the clinician returned the focus of the interview back to her mother and asked her to describe Amy's early history. She responded by describing Amy's early history of abuse and neglect. She was the product of an unwanted pregnancy and her mother had attempted to abort the pregnancy during her first trimester. After an uncomplicated delivery, her birth mother took Amy home but was depressed and unable to provide any consistent care for her daughter. For the next 6 months, Amy was cared for by numerous friends of her mother in her cluttered and unkempt apartment. During that time, her mother was in and out of the apartment and would go for weeks without contact with her daughter. Amy was finally removed from her mother's care by child protective services due to allegations of sexual and physical abuse. Over the course of 3 months, she was placed in two shelter homes before being placed with her prospective adoptive family.

Upon arriving at her adoptive placement, Amy was listless, underweight, and would "scream for hours on end." Bath time was particularly distressing, as she would scream uncontrollably and fight being placed in the bathtub. Her distress confused her adoptive mother, whose two children had always enjoyed their baths. Amy was unable to sleep through the night and would wake up several times a week with night terrors. Her mother was frustrated by her inability to soothe Amy and began to interpret this behavior as a sign of rejection. During the day, Amy was unable to engage in any quiet activities and after months of this stress, her mother was beginning to give up on engaging her in play. In fact, she was unable to think of any activities that Amy enjoyed and pointed out that she rarely, if ever, saw Amy laugh or smile. She added that her two biological children were frustrated by Amy's constant demands for their mother's attention, and were progressively disturbed by her bouts of unprovoked aggressive behavior. Furthermore, her marriage was starting to "fall apart" under the stress because her husband was resentful about the adoption and the negative impact Amy was having on their family. She was considering marital therapy but her husband felt that it was unnecessary given that the adoption was the sole source of the marital problems.

The observations of Amy's interactions with her mother and her response to the clinician's brief attempts at outreach, along with her early history of inconsistent caregiving, provided a significant amount of insight into Amy's emotional functioning and shed light on the status of the parent–child relationship. The mother's negative internal working model of Amy was alluded to in the first moments of the interview by her use of sarcasm to describe Amy's behavior as showing her "in her full glory," which was understood by the clinician as her attempt to convey the level of her distress with Amy's behavior. During the interview, she indicated that she was resentful of Amy and was losing patience with the high levels of aggression that were directed toward her and other family members. She was beginning to perceive Amy as an angry, emotionally distant child with whom she would never be able to form a loving relationship. This struggle was particularly disconcerting because it conflicted with her perception of herself as a warm, caring mother who had essentially saved Amy from a life of misery. Amy's "lack of appreciation" for being rescued left her mother feeling confused and dejected and was projected as confirmation of her perception of Amy as rejecting and unappreciative of her love and comfort.

Amy's behavior, however, told a different story. Her attempt to "swat" at the examiner when he attempted to engage her was interpreted by him as suggestive of an anxious and fearful, rather than an angry, oppositional little girl. Her traumatized caregiving history suggested that Amy had developed a negative working model of adults that had generalized to nearly anyone with whom she would come in contact. She had come to view herself as not worthy of love and affection and believed that she could not trust adults to engage with her in a nurturing manner. Consequently, she would "swat away" or reject adults before they would "inevitably" hurt or reject her.

Unfortunately, Amy's defensive style and use of aggression to keep others at bay was creating unintentional distance between her and her adoptive mother. While her mother, understandably, viewed the aggression negatively, she was unable to appreciate that the aggression was actually serving a dual purpose: an expression of anger and a simultaneous bid for protection. Amy, at the age of 2 and with limited speech, was unable to verbalize her needs adequately. In addition, given her early trauma history she had failed to learn how to discriminate her emotions; sadness, frustration, and anxiety were indistinguishable as separate emotional states. Thus, aggressive behavior assumed multiple meanings: she was angry with her mother for bringing her to a strange place but also sought protection. During the clinical interview, it was plausible that she bit her mother because she wanted to be picked up and protected from an anxiety-producing situation. In fact, the aggression did produce the desired result of being picked up and placed on her mother's lap. The clinician posited that if Amy had the necessary language skills she might have said, "Mommy, I'm terribly frightened of this man. You're mad at me but I need to be in your lap. Now! You're not listening and I'm getting scared! Please pick me up!" Thus, aggression was both a call for help and a vehicle for self-protection.

Utilizing an attachment framework, interview questions are designed to probe the attachment system by asking parents to describe positive times with the child, as well as painful and frustrating moments. Likewise, the parent is asked to describe events over the past several weeks when the child felt scared or frightened. The parent is then asked to talk about how the child responded as well as how the parent responded during the situation.

When asked to describe their positive time together, Amy's mother was unable to recall any positive experiences over the two weeks that preceded the interview. On the other hand, she provided a tremendous amount of detail about numerous power conflicts and uncontrollable temper outbursts that had occurred over this time. These had resulted in progressive isolation from public places and friends' homes. When asked how these problems were affecting their relationship she began to cry and stated that she was finding it progressively more difficult to experience any positive feelings for Amy, saying, "I'm ashamed to admit it but I really don't like her anymore." She added that there had been several incidents over the past weeks when Amy had fallen and hurt herself and, despite Amy's tears, she failed to attempt to soothe her. When asked about Amy's strengths and weaknesses she reported flatly that "Amy has lots of energy."

In summary, the interview findings indicated that Amy had suffered from physical and sexual abuse. Additionally, her experience with multiple caregivers had prevented her from developing trust in adults. Moreover, the lack of emotionally responsive caregiving had left her unable to differentiate her own emotions and without any strategies to self-soothe. Unfortunately, her early trauma was now generalized to most of the adults with whom she would come in contact; her only coping strategy was to use aggression and anger to keep others at bay. Her ability to explore her environment with any sense of play or positive emotion was virtually nonexistent. Finally, Amy was unable to engage positively with her adoptive family members, who were beginning to experience high levels of frustration with her.

Amy's adoptive mother portrayed her as an ungrateful, emotionally distant child, which made it difficult for her to respond to her daughter's pain. She needed help to understand, and respond to, Amy's high levels of anxiety. Additionally, treatment would need to help Amy's parents provide a secure base for Amy and become emotionally available for her when she needed to regulate her feelings.

While Amy had many treatment needs, for the purposes of this chapter I will address Amy's need to learn to trust adults and see them as being able to provide care and protection. The therapeutic preschool program also provided Amy with an opportunity to learn to engage positively with peers and adults and help her gain the skills needed to explore her environment. Additionally, she would receive speech and language therapy in order to help her learn to express her needs and emotions more effectively.

THE THERAPEUTIC PRESCHOOL INTERVENTION

Amy's mother embraced the idea of daily treatment for her daughter and was looking forward to 3 hours of "respite" each day. She accompanied Amy to her classroom on the first day, quickly told her good-bye, and stayed only minutes to watch her child adjust to her new surroundings. Amy accepted outreach from her teacher and, when prompted, waved good-bye to her mother while appearing helpless and resigned to the separation.

During Amy's initial weeks in the therapeutic preschool she would isolate herself in the corner, rarely played, and only occasionally tolerated contact with an adult. If the adults came too close she was quick to resort to her learned behavior of angrily scowling at them and swatting them away with her hands. Reluctantly, she learned to sit on the floor with her legs outstretched and tolerated rolling a ball between herself and one of the therapists. However, if they reached too far into her personal space she would physically withdraw and stop the play.

When Amy's peers approached her play space, she would physically shelter her toys, appearing fearful that they intended to take them away. She participated only minimally in group activities and avoided any contact with peers. On one occasion she began to cry when a child took a toy she was no longer using, and allowed herself to be picked up by her therapist. After several weeks, she began to show signs of seeking proximity toward this therapist when she needed help or support by looking toward her and physically moving a few steps in her direction.

Amy's lack of trust in adults was prioritized in her treatment planning. She needed to learn how to experience adults as a secure base and be able to turn to them for help when she felt frightened or hurt. In order to begin this process it was emphasized that staff should anticipate and respond to any self-care needs that she might exhibit. For example, by their approaching her and saying, "You look hungry, Amy, so I brought you some crackers," she might begin to experience adults as having the capacity to understand her needs and provide nurturing care. Positive, proactive outreach initiated by the adults on a daily basis set the stage for a reworking of her working model of self and others. That is, from Amy's perspective, if the adults could anticipate her needs they must be thinking about her, and if they were thinking about her she must be worthy of positive attention. Whenever she was even slightly injured, the staff would approach her and provide soothing, followed by emphasizing their concern for her safety.

As Amy became more relaxed with her interactions with the staff, they began to reflect her feelings on a broader scale. For example, when she wet herself they would say, "It doesn't feel good to be wet, let's go change so you'll feel better." When a child approached and she looked fearful they would reflect, "You were afraid that Johnny might hurt you or take your toy." After several months, Amy began using a wider vocabulary to express her feelings. In addition, as she learned to verbalize her feelings, her level of aggressive behavior started to subside.

During this period Amy continued to play with her toys in isolation and was quick to hover over them if any child approached her play space. This behavior was seen as a reflection of her negative internal working model of peers as wanting to threaten or attack her. The staff challenged this behavior whenever it occurred by interpreting, "You are afraid that Johnny is coming over to take your toy. But look! He is just walking over here slowly with a smile on his face. I think he wants to play." The two children would be supported in positive, cooperative play while the staff continued to interpret and reframe Amy's fear and negative view of peers.

Following 6 months of intensive, daily intervention, Amy began to initiate positive outreach to the adults and was less defensive when peers approached her play. She particularly enjoyed roughhousing with adults, and her fear of males was decreased when we discovered that she enjoyed giving "high five" by slapping their hands. When the males responded by feigning pain she would giggle with delight. Using a playful frame, Amy began to see that she could feel less threatened by, and simultaneously gain a sense of power over, her interactions with men. In addition, what had been a behavior designed to keep others at bay had become a positive means of engaging while simultaneously maintaining a sense of safety and positive boundaries within a relationship.

PARENT–CHILD PSYCHOTHERAPY

Parent–child psychotherapy is utilized as a parallel intervention with the therapeutic preschool program. By the end of the first 3 months of treatment Amy's adoptive parents were beginning to view her more positively. They observed her in the therapeutic preschool and were delighted by her increasingly positive peer interactions. Additionally, they began to model the empathic language used by the staff. However, they also expressed extreme distress with her continued aggressive behaviors at home. The couple disagreed about how to manage her behavior; Amy's mother was attempting to use time-outs in her room, while her father preferred spanking as an intervention. Additionally, their biological children were avoiding Amy because of her high levels of aggression and were constantly complaining to their parents about how much they disliked her. On one particularly upsetting evening, the oldest child actually verbalized that he was starting to wish he could move out and live with his friends.

The parent–child sessions focused on concerns about the daily bouts of aggression that Amy directed toward her mother. She bemoaned the fact that "Amy comes up to me for no reason and hits me. And it hurts!" The hitting and biting had failed to decrease despite lengthy time-outs in her bedroom. In fact, when Amy was sent to her room, her mother reported, she would scream, pound on the door, and then start to destroy her toys. Upon hearing the destruction, her mother would enter the room, place Amy harshly on her bed, tell her to "stop it!" and storm out. This usually resulted in Amy crying uncontrollably for over 5 minutes before storming out of her room and sulking in a corner within view of her mother. This scenario was repeated numerous times each day.

In one of the parent–child sessions, when Amy's mother arrived she was so emotionally fatigued that she was unable to join Amy in any play. Amy played briefly with the toys but primarily scattered them about the floor, which was terribly irritating to her mother. When she yelled at Amy to pick up the toys before taking anything else out, Amy walked over and bit her on the hand. When she screeched in pain, Amy's mother interpreted her daughter's smile as an indicator of delight in her pain.

The therapist reflected that when Amy was angry with her mother she would bite her so that her mother would become angry, which was actually her attempt to help them share the experience of being angry. That is, Amy's behavior effectively communicated, "I'm angry and now you're feeling as angry as me!" In order to move beyond the cycle of anger, it was important for Amy to begin to acquire an ability to empathize with others in order to enhance the parent–child attachment. To do so, her mother was encouraged to grimace and dramatize the pain that Amy inflicted when she hit or bit. Moments later, Amy walked up to her mother and hit her on the leg. Her mother responded by clutching her knee and looking terribly pained. Amy stopped, looked at her mother with a rather stunned expression, and then walked up to her and patted her softly. While she had learned to develop a high level of defensiveness in response to anger, Amy was ready at this point in time to respond with care and comfort when she recognized pain. Over the next few months, Amy's aggression toward her mother, though it persisted, decreased considerably.

Amy's parent's, however, continued to disagree about how to manage her remaining temper outbursts. Her father continued to rely on spanking as an intervention while her mother was frustrated by the need to "constantly drag her off to time out" and reported that time-out seemed to be ineffective in bringing about any changes in her behavior. The concept of "time in" (see Powell et al., Chapter 7, this volume, on the Circle of Security) was shared with her as a more attachment-focused alternative. The concept of "time in" is based on the observation that when children are emotionally dysregulated, they need proximity to the caregiver rather than distance. Thus, she was encouraged to remain close to Amy during her temper outbursts and provide physical comfort and reassurance that once she calmed down they could fix the problem. If Amy responded with any level of aggression, her mother was encouraged to move away from Amy while saying, "I want to stay safe. But I will be right here so that I can help you as soon as you calm down." If Amy continued to escalate, her mother was encouraged to move farther away or even say, "I'll be in the [next room] but I will be listening to you and as soon as you're calm I'll be right back." Through this process, Amy learned to view her mother as a secure base who could reliably provide comfort and nurturing care. As she learned to regulate her feelings, her destructive behaviors significantly decreased. Whereas "time out" in her room had escalated her anxiety and sense of isolation, through "time in" Amy learned to be less frightened by her own feelings of distress.

As Amy's violence decreased, her mother was beginning to enjoy spending more time with her. This was reflected in their play during the therapy sessions, as she was able to begin to show delight in Amy's exploration of the toys and respond positively when Amy shared her little creations with her. On one occasion Amy began to show signs of frustration when her wooden tower kept falling down. Amy suddenly turned to her mother and said, "Mommy! I need help!" Amy had never before expressed the need for her mother and it was a significant turning point in their relationship. Amy's mother could now assist her daughter in exploring the environment and, when needed, Amy was able to turn to her mother for help and comfort.

The sibling relationships continued to be marked by conflict, however, and Amy's mother was distressed by the children's constant conflict during play. They were also engaging her in what she termed "chronic tattle-telling." Using the attachment framework, the tattle-telling was reframed as their need for her to be a secure base. That is, they were turning to her for assistance because they were frustrated or frightened. She was encouraged to respond by praising them for coming for help and then more actively helping the children work out a solution. Weeks later, though still fatigued by their need for her support, she was also pleased to see the children showing signs of getting along. She also pointed out that she liked being needed by Amy as well as by her two boys.

CLOSING COMMENTS

Amy's early history created negative working models for how she could expect to be treated and, as well, what she could expect from her caregivers. Her lack of verbal strategies forced her to rely on aggression to communicate fear and anger but, in addition, aggression was used to convey a desperate need for protection. The therapeutic preschool program was able to provide a setting in which Amy could safely learn to rely on adults for comfort when she was hurt or frustrated. She also learned to appreciate that adults could support her as she learned to explore her environment. As Amy began to view adults more positively she slowly generalized this to home and became less aggressive and more affectionate toward her family. Through the use of parent–child psychotherapy sessions, her mother learned to reinterpret Amy's behaviors and respond with more empathy and nurturance. Utilizing attachment-based treatment strategies the two treatment modalities were used to challenge Amy's negative internal working models, which enabled her to learn to enjoy relationships with her parents, her adoptive siblings, and several peers in her therapeutic preschool group. During a 1-year follow-up session, her mother reported continued frustration with some of Amy's challenging behaviors but, in general, was able to state that she fully enjoyed being Amy's mother. The three children were described as engaging in bouts of conflict that she described as "typical sibling rivalry" and Amy was functioning positively in a regular preschool program.

ACKNOWLEDGMENTS

I would like to thank my colleague Sandi Isaacson, PhD, for her careful review of this chapter and for her insights regarding the application of attachment theory to clinical practice.

REFERENCES

Bowlby, J. (1982). *Attachment* (2nd ed.). New York: Basic Books. (Original work published 1969)

Bowlby, J. (1988). *A secure base: Parent–child attachment and healthy human development*. New York: Basic Books.

Bretherton, I. (2005). In pursuit of the internal working model construct and its relevance to attachment relationships. In K. E. Grossman, K. Grossman, & E. Waters (Eds.), *Attachment from infancy to adulthood: The major longitudinal studies* (pp. 13–47). New York: Guilford Press.

Carlson, E. A., & Sroufe, L. A. (1995). Contributions of attachment theory to developmental psychopathology. In D. Cicchetti & D. J. Cohen (Eds.), *Developmental psychopathology* (Vol. 1, pp. 581–617). New York: Wiley.

Cassidy, J., & Koback, R. R. (1988). Avoidance and its relation to other defensive processes. In J. Belsky & T. Nezworski (Eds.), *Clinical implications of attachment* (pp. 300–326). Hillsdale, NJ: Erlbaum.

Cicchetti, D., Ganiban, J., & Barnett, D. (1991). Contributions from the study of high-risk populations to understanding the development of emotion regulation. In J. Garber & K. A. Dodge (Eds.), *The development of emotion regulation and dysregulation* (pp. 15–48). New York: Cambridge University Press.

Fonagy, P. (2001). *Attachment theory and psychoanalysis*. New York: Other Press.

Greenberg, M., Spelz, M., DeKlyen, M., & Endriga, M. (1991). Attachment security in preschoolers with and without externalizing behavior problems: a replication. *Developmental Psychopathology, 3*, 413–430.

Hirshberg, L. M. (1996). History-making, not history-taking: Clinical interviews with infants and their families. In S. J. Meisels & E. Fenichel (Eds.), *New visions for the developmental assessment of infants and young children* (pp. 85–124). Washington, DC: Zero to Three Press.

Lieberman, A. F. (2004). Child–parent psychotherapy: A relationship-based approach to the treatment of mental health disorders in infancy and early childhood. In A. J. Sameroff, S. C. McDonough, & K. L. Rosenblum (Eds.), *Treating parent–infant relationship problems: Strategies for intervention* (pp. 97–122). New York: Guilford Press.

Pawl, J. H. (1995). The therapeutic relationship as human connectedness: Being held in another's mind. *Zero to Three, 15*(4), 1–5.

Plenk, A. M. (1993). *Helping young children at risk: A psycho-educational approach*. Westport, CT: Praeger.

Sameroff, A. J. (2004). Ports of entry and the dynamics of mother–infant interventions. In A. J. Sameroff, S. C. McDonough, & K. L. Rosenblum (Eds.), *Treating parent–infant relationship problems: Strategies for intervention* (pp. 3–28). New York: Guilford Press.

Sroufe, L. A. (1995). *Emotional development: The organization of emotional life in the early years*. New York: Cambridge University Press.

Sroufe, L. A. (2005). Attachment and development: A prospective, longitudinal study from birth to adulthood. *Attachment and Human Development, 7*(4), 349–367.

Steele, H., & Steele, M. (2005). Understanding and resolving emotional conflict: The London Parent–Child Project. In K. E. Grossman, K. Grossman, & E. Waters (Eds.), *Attachment from infancy to adulthood: The major longitudinal studies* (pp. 137–164). New York: Guilford Press.

Waters, E., & Sroufe, L. A. (1983). Social competence as a developmental construct. *Developmental Review, 3*, 79–97.

Winnicott, D. W. (1965). *The maturational process and the facilitating environment: Studies in the theory of emotional development*. New York: International University Press.

CHAPTER NINE

Disorganized Mother, Disorganized Child

The Mentalization of Affective Dysregulation and Therapeutic Change

ARIETTA SLADE

Despite its initial hostility to attachment theory (Holmes, 1995), psychoanalysis has over the past 15 years gradually come to accept the importance and validity of Bowlby and his colleagues' groundbreaking contributions (see Slade, 1999a, 1999b, and 2000, for a review). The integration of attachment theory within the psychoanalytic mainstream is due largely to the seminal efforts of Mary Main, Peter Fonagy, and their colleagues, whose work has galvanized many aspects of dynamic theory and practice (Fonagy, 2000, 2001; Fonagy et al., 1995; Fonagy, Gergely, Jurist, & Target, 2002; Fonagy & Target, 1996, 1998; Hesse & Main, 2000; Main, 1995; Main & Hesse, 1990; Main, Kaplan, & Cassidy, 1985).

Nevertheless, while the essential concepts of attachment *theory* have been easy for clinicians to embrace, as they are largely concordant with many of the basic assumptions of contemporary psychoanalysis

(Mitchell, 1999), the methods and implications of attachment *research* have been more difficult for dynamically oriented psychotherapists to integrate into practice. In particular, psychoanalytic clinicians have found it challenging to locate the vitality and clinical utility in the concept of *attachment classification*, as this notion—absolutely central to much of attachment research—is seen as reducing and oversimplifying complex mental phenomena.

In this chapter, I am returning to a theme that has interested me for some time, namely the relevance of attachment classification specifically, and attachment theory more broadly, to clinical thinking and practice (see too Slade, 1999b, 2004a, 2004b, in press). I have for the past 25 years worked both as an attachment researcher and psychoanalytic psychologist; thus, my understanding of how attachment representations and attendant mentalizing capacities develop over time and function to regulate affect and relationships has deepened at the same time that my practice as a clinician has evolved. Thus, attachment organization and reflective functioning are essential to the way I think about and work with patients, just as are other aspects of psychoanalytic theory and practice. They are not opposing but, rather, complementary constructs.

In this chapter, I am going to focus on how my individual work with a long-term psychotherapy patient was influenced by my seeing her as disorganized/unresolved in relation to attachment. This construct, first introduced by Mary Main and Judith Solomon (Main & Solomon,1980) and later elaborated by Main and Hesse (Hesse & Main, 2000; Main & Hesse, 1990), describes the most potentially pathological of the three insecure categories (the others being avoidant/dismissive and resistant/preoccupied); as a function of its roots in traumatic experience (Lyons-Ruth & Jacobvitz, 1999; Main & Hesse, 1990) it is also typified by dramatic lapses in mentalization and reflective functioning (Fonagy et al., 2002). Such patients are relatively common in latter-day clinical practice; they can also be quite difficult to treat and productively engage in treatment.

I begin with a brief review of the central assumptions of attachment theory, which will serve as a backdrop to the construct of disorganized attachment. I then describe the essential aspects of this attachment classification, using an actual mother–infant interaction vignette as illustration. I then use these constructs as the backdrop for a discussion of an ongoing psychotherapy case. In this way, I hope to draw helpful links between infant observation, attachment classification, and adult treatment.

ATTACHMENT AND CARESEEKING:
A BRIEF OVERVIEW

Bowlby, writing as an early object relations theorist, suggested that the baby is born with a predisposition to seek care from its caregivers (Bowlby, 1969, 1973, 1980). Because his survival depends upon it, the infant is biologically programmed to seek the care of someone older and wiser—an attachment figure. The child seeks the caregiver's security and protection for many reasons, but particularly in moments when he or she is frightened or in danger.[1] Thus, careseeking often takes place in moments of high affective arousal, arousal that is then—optimally—regulated by the caregiver (K. Lyons-Ruth, personal communication, April 9, 2003; Lyons-Ruth, Bronfman, & Atwood, 1999). And by virtue of her role as regulator and container of that affect, the mother's response to the infant's affect becomes a part of that affective experience (see too Fairbairn, 1952; Stern, 1985; Tronick & Weinberg, 1997).

Children quickly figure out how to seek care in a way that will minimally disrupt their vital relationship to their caregiver. One of the things they must learn in this process is which affects are tolerable to caregivers, and which are not. They learn this via the repetition—again and again—of a particular relational drama around the expression of careseeking. Over time, their efforts to regulate their affects in such a way as to maintain their primary relationships become organized into what attachment theorists refer to as attachment patterns, namely organized or characteristic ways of seeking care from and preserving closeness with the caregiver. Psychoanalysts would consider these primitive efforts to protect the self from intolerable affects to be early signs of defense and identification. But in the earliest months and years of life, these efforts arise first in the effort to protect the other (Winnicott, 1965). And it is these ways of protecting the other and ultimately the self from affects that disrupt careseeking and caregiving that become internal representations of attachment or—in analytic terms—central aspects of psychic structure.

---

[1] I do not mean to suggest that moments of joy, pleasure, and reciprocity between parent and child are not equally crucial in the development of the child's sense of self. Indeed, in situations such as those I describe here, memories of joy and of truly reciprocal exchange are all but absent. Nevertheless, such moments are not typically those in which the child seeks the parent's care and protection, which is what I am focusing on here.

Because the survival of infants is dependent upon success in their careseeking efforts, these are psychologically and physically critical events. Without proximal care and containment, infants cannot function (Bowlby, 1969, 1973, 1982, 1988), and cannot learn (Brazelton & Cramer, 1990). Thus, they must shape themselves (and their experience of affect and arousal) to ensure that their needs are met. They *must* obtain care, at whatever cost to their functioning. Aspects of self-experience, and especially affective experience, that preclude the maintenance of attachment relationships are disavowed, reversed, fragmented, or dissociated. Knowing, thinking, and feeling emerge within the context of maintaining vital connections, and of continuing to exist in the other's mind. Children quickly learn what kinds of thoughts and emotions can be borne within the context of their primary attachments. It is within his or her earliest relationships that a child's core sense of self in relation to arousal, to affect, and to careseeking is laid down.

Attachment classifications provide us a way of describing the dynamics of arousal regulation and the subjective experience of careseeking. A secure baby is one who can comfortably go to the caregiver when frightened, sad, or angry, while an insecure baby alters these states to fit the needs of the caregiver. In adults, these same patterns are reflected in the way an adult regulates affect within the structure of narrative. Early moments of regulation live on in the structure of speech, of thought, and of affects (Main et al., 1985). When we listen carefully to the contradictions, dysfluencies, and disruptions in narrative, we are witnessing the representation in language and thought of early dyadic experiences of disrupted careseeking and dysregulation.

ANAROSA AND SOPHIA

I begin with a brief description of the interaction between AnaRosa and her 4-month-old baby, Sophia. This interactive moment will then serve as a backdrop for introducing the construct of disorganized attachment

AnaRosa had her baby just after she turned age 18. She had a long history of trauma, including the death of her father, placement in foster care, and sexual abuse by a relative. AnaRosa was a participant in the Minding the Baby program (Slade, Sadler, & Mayes, 2005; Slade et al., 2005); she entered the program in the second trimester of her pregnancy. As part of our research, we saw AnaRosa and her baby in a standard face-to-face interaction setting when the baby was 4 months old.

AnaRosa was asked to interact with her daughter as she ordinarily would, but without toys or other objects; they were simply to engage with one another *en face*. AnaRosa found this instruction very difficult: her baby was just waking up from a nap, she was (we learned later) hungry, and AnaRosa felt pressured to "perform" for the camera. What resulted was an alarming interaction in which AnaRosa intruded upon Sophia's physical and visual space in an extremely aggressive way for nearly 20 minutes. She poked, she loomed, she slapped in a playful but very rough way, and she mocked Sophia's distress. The baby looked stunned, and attempted in a variety of ways to regulate her mother's insistent and overwhelming approach. At moments she looked away and seemed almost dissociated, at others she looked actively frightened and blinked her eyes as if trying to blot her mother out, at others she fussed mildly, and at others she struggled to placate with a dazed half-smile. Often all of these efforts were taking place at once. What was most striking was that she rarely fully broke gaze with her mother; she could not take the "alone" and integrative time so vital in any *en face* interaction (Brazelton & Cramer, 1990) because she could not risk letting her mother out of her sight. AnaRosa missed many of the baby's cues, notably her fear, her dysregulation, and her intentions. It was a profoundly disrupted interaction in which normal reciprocity and pacing were entirely absent, and was painful to watch.[2]

This interaction captures beautifully the complex issues surrounding the regulation of fear in the attachment relationship when the mother is frightening to the baby. Ordinarily, children seek comfort from their caregiver when they are afraid; this is a prime reason for the child's seeking proximity and care. In the case of AnaRosa and Sophia, the mother—who felt both helpless in relation to her baby because she could not engage her in the way she thought she should, and hostile toward her because Sophia was potentially exposing her failure—was at once the source of and the solution to the baby's fear (Lyons-Ruth et al., 1999; Main & Hesse, 1990). Sophia was faced with an irresolvable paradox: the person she was afraid of was also the person she had to rely on to assuage and regulate her fear. The paradox was all over the baby's face: Should she signal fear or pleasure? Was she safer just zoning out?

---

[2]The good news is that some 10 months later, after regular participation in the intervention, AnaRosa and her baby looked infinitely better than they had at this early assessment. Most importantly, Sophia was not disorganized in relation to attachment at 1 year.

These sorts of interactions form the basis, in infancy, for the development of *disorganized* attachment, which can be measured at 1 year using Ainsworth's Strange Situation (Ainsworth, Blehar, Waters, & Wall, 1978; Lyons-Ruth & Jacobvitz, 1999). Disorganization refers to several aspects of the attachment representation. First, because the caregiver is both frightened by and frightening to the baby, he or she cannot develop an organized and coherent way of seeking care from the mother. Fear overwhelms the normal functioning of the attachment system, disrupting proximity seeking and contact maintenance. Directly approaching the mother risks evoking her fearful or frightening behavior; thus, children who are disorganized in relation to attachment establish contact in odd, stereotypic, or contradictory ways. Often this involves entering a dissociative state, such that attachment needs and strivings are dissociated from consciousness, and from the interaction. What Lyons-Ruth and her colleagues (1999) suggest is that the experience of being frightened of or frightening to the caregiver gives rise to the experience of feeling helpless or hostile *in relation* to the caregiver; as a result, attachment relationships and attachment representations become organized along and around a helpless–hostile continuum.

Optimally, playful (or any other sort of) engagement with the mother leads the child over time to identify his own internal states, as they are first *re*-presented to him by the mother within the framework of the interaction. "Anxiety, for example, is for the infant a confusing mixture of physiological changes, ideas, and behaviors. When the mother reflects, or mirrors, the child's anxiety, this perception organizes the child's experience and he now 'knows' what he is feeling" (Fonagy et al., 2002). It is in this very concrete way that she serves as a container and organizer of the child's early emotional experiences. For dyads like AnaRosa and Sophia, however, the child's feelings and needs—for affiliation, comfort, regulation, and the like—are not acknowledged by the mother, presumably because they are too evocative and painful for her (Lyons-Ruth et al., 1999). In this instance, they stimulated her aggression and scorn. For Sophia, contemplating her mother's mind involved contemplating her mother's hatred and rage. Thus, rather than contemplate and ultimately internalize these distorted and terrifying representations, she was left little choice other than to dissociate and fragment her awareness of her mother's or her own mental states. It is in these situations, suggests Fonagy, that children develop an "alien" (Fonagy et al., 2002) self to ensure survival. This alien self reflects an identification with the caregiver's self states, because one's own cannot be acknowledged and known within the context of the relationship. In the vignette I just described, it is possible to see Sophia's alien or false self (Winnicott, 1965) in formation.

In the case of disorganized attachment, the child gradually identifies with the parent's helpless and/or hostile states of mind, states of mind that emerge as a function of the parent's experience of being frightened (helpless) or frightening (hostile) in relation to the child. These sorts of identifications likely form the basis of the controlling/punitive and help-less/inhibited orientations of the school-age disorganized child (George & Solomon, 1998; Lyons-Ruth & Jacobvitz, 1999), and may evolve into the competing representational strategies that are the hallmark of disor-ganized attachment in adults. Competing representational strategies are marked by "discontinuity or dissociation of mental contents at the level of mental representation" (Lyons-Ruth et al., 1999, p. 34). Thus, when asked to describe their early relationship experiences—especially the experience of loss, abuse, or other attachment-related trauma—the dis-course of disorganized adults is disrupted, characterized by lapses in rea-soning and monitoring, as well as by a range of other narrative oddities and dysfluencies, all of which serve to fragment awareness of the painful mental states associated with trauma (Main & Hesse, 1990).

This internal disorganization has a direct impact on the interaction with the child. Just as the parent cannot repair the splits in his or her own mental representations, he or she cannot repair the disruptions in his or her interaction with the child that result from his or her own competing and conflicting self-states. Because the child's frightened responses evoke her own "past losses or fear-evoking experiences," the parent restricts her "conscious attention to the infant's fear-related cues. . . . The more pervasive these restrictions on the parent's conscious attention and responsiveness, the more the parent's need to regulate her own negative arousal will take precedence over the infant's concomitant need for a soothing response to his or her attachment-related communi-cations" (Lyons-Ruth et al., p. 38). Thus, AnaRosa could not process her child's alarm and fear, as she was herself angry at feeling pressured to perform and "play," something she felt quite unequipped to do.

CYNTHIA AND LUISA

I would like to use this brief description of disorganized attachment as a backdrop for talking about Cynthia, a patient I have been seeing twice weekly for the past 2 years. Cynthia is an attractive woman in her 40s who came to see me at the recommendation of her daughter's psychiatrist, Dr. Jenkins. Thirteen-year-old Luisa was being seen for a range of attentional and behavioral problems. Due to the disrupted relationship between Cynthia and Luisa, who was adopted, the psychiatrist suspected that "attachment" problems were at the root of some of Luisa's difficulties. Dr. Jenkins felt that she could better address Luisa's issues if Cynthia had a better handle on her own very complex feelings about mothering her daughter.

The Opening Session: The Traumatized and Traumatizing Caregiver

Cynthia arrived at my office casually but elegantly dressed, perfectly put together. She was pleasant and almost deferential. But my sense of her orderliness shifted rapidly as she began to tell me her story. This did not have to do with the details of her life story (which were, admittedly, very painful to hear) but with the way she told the story. Many things came out in a rush. She first told me about how she was referred to me. She seemed aggrieved by the suggestion that her own issues might play a role in Luisa's symptoms; this had obviously been shameful for her. She was upset by Dr. Jenkins's suggestion that—given both her current situation and past history—she must be "very angry." "I'm not angry!" she exclaimed to me. She was also understandably confused by the recommendation that she and her daughter see an "attachment therapist," who encouraged the child to describe her thoughts and feelings about her adoption and her birth mother while Cynthia held Luisa on her lap.[3] She then told me about her divorce, which was in litigation for 3 years and rivaled some of the most public and highly publicized divorces for its cruelty and impropriety. Adding to her sense of betrayal and shame was the fact that her husband had immediately remarried, to a socially prominent woman whose social circles regularly overlapped with Cynthia's. There were no opportunities for emotional escape or distance in her life.

Next she laid out for me the barest outlines of a childhood filled with abuse, alcoholism, and unremitting violence and fear. Her father—a highly successful lawyer—was both an alcoholic and mentally ill, and

---

[3]Space does not permit a full discussion of this aspect of her daughter's treatment, which I found highly problematic and likely—given the dynamics described here—quite unhelpful.

viciously abused his six children throughout their childhoods. Her mother, also an alcoholic, was also abused by her husband, and failed to protect Cynthia or her siblings from their father. And while little of her mother's cruelty and narcissism was revealed during this initial session, it has become clear over the course of our work that her mother's envy, meanness, and readiness to humiliate and shame was as damaging as her father's more overt abuse. Her parents divorced when she was a teenager. She currently has a difficult and often painful relationship with her mother, who is quite elderly, emotionally fragile, but mean and shaming as ever. Cynthia is in touch with only one of her siblings. She has strong evidence that one of her brothers sexually abused her older (biological) daughter, Emma, who is about to finish college.

Emma was 4 when Luisa was adopted a year after Cynthia nearly died as the result of complications during a second, unsuccessful pregnancy. Subsequent surgeries left her infertile. Thus, Luisa's adoption must be seen within the context of yet another unresolved, terrifying trauma.

I felt overwhelmed by the time Cynthia left at the end of our initial consultation—a little bit like AnaRosa's daughter. The story had come out all at once, and I felt the chaos and violence deeply, almost as if I had been assaulted by it myself. I was disrupted and disoriented. On the one hand, I could use constructs like primitive object relations, projective identification, PTSD, borderline personality disorder, or pathological narcissism to organize my thinking about Cynthia. And to some extent, I did. On the other hand, I found it more helpful to think of her as someone disorganized in relation to attachment.

The Markers of Disorganized Attachment

There were numerous signs that Cynthia was both disorganized in relation to her own parents as well as disorganized/unresolved in her caregiving.[4] First was her history of *unresolved* trauma, told in an

---

[4]It will not be possible to fully discuss the obvious fact that Luisa is herself likely also disorganized in relation to attachment. Indeed, this would explain what the psychiatrist was responding to in referring the dyad for attachment therapy. It would also explain a range of Luisa's contradictory behaviors in relation to her mother. Interestingly, Luisa, like many adopted children, has the desire to seek out her birth mother. The split maternal representation (her "lost" mother being her "good" mother) is another indicator of Luisa's disorganized status, specifically her concretely representing the disorganized paradox by carrying two mothers in her mind.

unmetabolized and yet highly charged way. The most significant clue to the fact that she had not resolved the multiple traumas of her childhood was the incoherent quality of her narrative, suggesting the failure to organize, represent, or mentalize a number of aspects of her childhood experience. While incoherence is not in and of itself a marker of disorganization, the lapses in discourse that typified Cynthia's narrative are. While the story was horrible, Cynthia's affect was one of a court reporter, reciting the facts without apparent affect. Although she punctuated her story with looks of horror and resignation, the story did not feel as if she were experiencing it in a real way. The story felt canned, and the affect dissociated. Adding to my sense of her need to isolate herself from affect was her referring to her former husband as "the father," Emma as "my daughter," and Luisa as "the kid." Rarely would she call them by name.

Her narrative was incoherent in other ways as well. It was both too long (quantity) as well as tangential, overly detailed, and yet surprisingly noncommunicative (quality). She had difficulty collaborating with me as a listener. She discharged, I received. It was as if Cynthia was so disconnected from her story that all she could do was assault me with it; this was how she told me what it was like to be her. Traumatized individuals cannot easily think about what they are saying, and so the story loses its direction as they struggle not to think the unthinkable or feel the intolerable. The only time that her affect seemed genuine was when she described her surprise and humiliation at Dr. Jenkins's suggestion that she might be "very angry," and that her daughter had "attachment problems." While we would later come to recognize that—as a function of the dynamics of her early childhood relationships—humiliation was a very potent trigger for her, at this early point in the work she could not reconcile Dr. Jenkins's observation with the realities of her own story, or with her difficulties mothering her daughter. There were few indices of either metacognitive monitoring (Main, 1991) or mentalization (Fonagy et al., 1995). Cynthia had learned to isolate herself from the terrifying minds of others as a way of surviving; in this way, her parents, siblings, and children could not be (and were not) real people with real minds (Fonagy et al., 2002). In fact, the degree to which she really could not read people or their motives explained—in part—the poor choices she'd made in choosing men, as well as the multiple ways in which she had difficulty making sense of her daughter.

The clue to the fact that her affect was—despite myriad efforts to dissociate it—still highly live and disorganizing for her was my experience in the countertransference: I felt overwhelmed, mildly fearful, and somewhat dissociated at the end of our first session. It was as if I became the frightened, overwhelmed baby, and she became the dissociated aggressor. After our first session I must have felt what she experienced as a child, exposed to chronic violence and ongoing dysregulation, continuously fragmenting attention as a means of protecting any sense of self, and placating the terrifying caregiver. Unable to integrate feelings of vulnerability and fear, or to acknowledge the degree to which she felt violated and assaulted, she instead identified with the aggressor (Fraiberg, 1980). Her unintegrated anger was indeed palpable. We were like AnaRosa and Sophia, the traumatized mother frightening and overwhelming her baby as she had been traumatized and overwhelmed herself (Lyons-Ruth et al., 1999).

Thus, in my initial sessions with her, I began to hear and *experience* the signs of disorganized attachment. This meant, very concretely, that I began to think of her as someone whose relationships and internal life were characterized by the effort to manage the competing self and relational states of helplessness (triggered by feelings of fear and shame) and hostility (Lyons-Ruth et al., 1999). To do this—like Sophia in her interaction with AnaRosa—Cynthia relied primarily upon dissociation and other primitive attempts at organization and control. When these failed, she was herself frightening and rageful. Experiencing her in this way allowed me to imagine her as a child, assaulted and disrupted at every turn, but forced to regulate fear and other powerful negative affects without losing whatever contact was possible with her traumatizing parents. It also helped me imagine what it might be like to be Luisa.

This way of thinking about Cynthia guided not only my clinical formulation but also the way I spoke to her, the metaphors I used, the issues I focused on, and my overall therapeutic stance. What I hope to make clear in the following sections is that successful and productive therapeutic exchanges were those in which we engaged around moments of high-intensity arousal as a means of integrating mutually contradictory self-states, such that Cynthia could find a way to balance and ultimately regulate states of helpless withdrawal, dissociation, and frightening rage. This was possible only within the context of a positive and sustaining therapeutic relationship in which I steadily mentalized these contradictory self-states, remaining attuned to both their fluctuations and triggers.

The Work with Cynthia

Over the course of the past 2 years, Cynthia and I have generally talked about four things: her relationship with Luisa, her relationship with her mother, her ongoing feelings about the divorce and its aftermath, and her (now ended) relationship with the man she'd become involved with at the end of her marriage. In this chapter, I am going to focus primarily on the work we have done around her relationship with Luisa. It is here that the most dramatic changes have been apparent, largely as a function of the fact that things are often very "hot" with her daughter; thus, when we are discussing Luisa, we are often discussing moments when Cynthia has felt dysregulated and enraged, giving us an opportunity to vividly encounter the kinds of self–object affect representations that are evoked by experiences of dysregulation. Also, I think the desire to right things with Luisa has motivated her tremendously, and allowed her to see things about herself that she might otherwise avoid. Cynthia genuinely wishes *not* to repeat her own experience of being mothered in a rageful and punitive way. This is a crucial impetus to genuine change.

From the start of treatment, Cynthia has struggled to find a balance in her relationship with and representation of Luisa between the two states of mind that exemplify the disorganized paradox, helplessness and hostility (Lyons-Ruth, et al., 1999). Her most comfortable position is somewhere between the two, manifest in the somewhat dissociated talk that is hard to penetrate and seems quite false. This is when she is talking about or objectifying Luisa, calling her "the kid" and describing her behavior in a cut-off, sometimes almost theatrical way. Within the context of our work together, I have named this way of talking "on remote"; using this term, I can signal her shift into dissociation within the course of a session. Up until she began treatment, this was likely Cynthia's only way of keeping feelings of helplessness or rage at bay.

While Cynthia's rage at Luisa was the aspect of their relationship that was most palpable to all concerned (Cynthia, Luisa, Dr. Jenkins, the attachment therapist, and me), I came to see that these feelings were largely triggered when Cynthia felt fearful or humiliated in relation to Luisa (the flip side of her hostile stance). Luisa is not an easy child to love or to mother; she is disorganized, needy, self-absorbed, and wrapped up in things that seem to Cynthia incomprehensible. Like many children with ADHD,[5] Luisa finds things that interest her, takes them apart, hides them, loses them, and the like. She will then "lie" about it, trying to avoid the inevitable consequences; indeed, much of her lying seems a misguided attempt to forestall her mother's rages. Luisa's impulsivity, unpredictability, and often very chaotic behavior would arouse tremendous fear in Cynthia, because—just as was the case in her childhood—unpredictability means grave danger. Thus, when Luisa would "surprise" her, or act out—even mildly—Cynthia would become enraged. At these times, she could be cruel and punitive to her daughter, and would sometimes frightens her. She would come in and regale me with the "awful" things Luisa had done (and indeed Luisa was quite provocative), and then describe in a cut-off and rationalized way her own responses, which ranged from telling Luisa that she could go live with her father (who they both knew will not have her) to saying that she, Cynthia, had "had it" and was just going to go off and live by herself. She would often berate Luisa for "deliberately" and knowingly lying and manipulating. She would withhold affection and sometimes punish her too impulsively. When I would see Luisa in the waiting room, she indeed looked somewhat stunned and dissociated.

Cynthia found Luisa's lying utterly humiliating. For her the feeling of being marginalized (disrespected, ignored, manipulated, exploited) by her daughter was deeply shaming, for it implied to her that she meant nothing to Luisa, and affirmed her helplessness and the futility of her signaling anything to her daughter. Finally, it made clear to her that she was a bad mother (why else would Luisa ignore her?), just like her own mother. In effect, Luisa's acting out exposed Cynthia's flaws as a mother. Each of Luisa's provocations was a narcissistic injury, bringing with it the full fury of Cynthia's narcissistic rage, as well as the effort to turn Luisa into the helpless victim rather than (as Cynthia perceived her) the hostile attacker. This dynamic captures clearly the helpless–hostile relational diathesis described by Lyons-Ruth and colleagues (1999); when Cynthia felt helpless in the face of what she imagined to be Luisa's hostility, she endeavored to make Luisa feel helpless by herself becoming hostile. Once projected onto Luisa, this helplessness would ultimately lead to her feeling hostile.

---

[5] I fully recognize that this diagnosis serves as a shorthand for many types of regulatory disorders (Barkley, 1997), including those that are largely the consequence of disrupted or disorganized relationships.

Cynthia has an abiding fantasy that someday her children will feel about her the way she feels about her mother. This fantasy is deeply entrenched and even after over 2 years of treatment is barely open to examination. It is nearly impossible for Cynthia to see the difference between her relationship with her daughters and her mother's relationship with her own children. She is so deeply identified with her mother's helplessness and rage, identified both with the terrorist and the terrorized, that she cannot envision a different sort of outcome.

Because Cynthia experienced Luisa through the template of her own striated inner world, and her struggle with contradictory self-states, she had little abiding sense of her daughter's inner life as separate from hers. In the beginning of treatment she could not see Luisa outside of the context of her own helpless–hostile conundrum: Luisa is either the attacker or the weak victim of Cynthia's attack. A parent who did not fear mentalization might recognize that Luisa has her own reasons for doing what she does (among them to provoke her mother and bolster her own fragile self-esteem); however, each time Luisa acted out, Cynthia felt personally humiliated. She saw Luisa in terms of her own projections, and thus described her in terms of her behavior (bad) and not her internal experience (Slade, in press). When Cynthia became more able to imagine reasons for Luisa's behavior *that had nothing to do with her*, she became less angry and more sympathetic.[6] Indeed, she has in recent months begun to genuinely appreciate just how bad Luisa feels about herself, and to understand some of her (mis)behavior as a sign of her feeling unworthy and unlovable.

Over the course of our 2 years of work together, it has become more and more possible for Cynthia to move out of the dichotomy between frightened and frightening and find a way to remain in the room while at the same time regulating her rage. In these moments she can be quite authentic and engaged with her inner experience. When she finds this middle ground with Luisa, she can be real and present. It is in these moments that Cynthia can begin to experience herself as spontaneous, regulated, regulating, and loving. She can feel very directly the impact this has had on Luisa, who is generally much more spontaneous,

---

[6]I do not for a moment wish to overlook the fact that Luisa is indeed acting out the role of perpetrator and attacker at times; she, too, has internalized the paradox of the disorganized state of mind. Thus, the paradox that exists in Cynthia's mind also exists in Luisa's and in the dynamics of their tormented and tormenting relationship.

affectionate, and calm, and her "odd" behaviors more modulated; she is also less frightened by her mother.

The work with Cynthia has, of course, had many aspects, but I will mention a few that seem particularly important in view of her disorganized attachment status. Because moments of high-intensity affect, particularly fear, are so disorganizing for Cynthia, their appearance in the treatment provides crucial ports of entry and opportunities for reorganization (or in her case, organization) and change. My serving as a mentalizing other is vital (Fonagy et al., 2002), as it would be in any treatment, but because she easily slides into "remote," the most productive moments occur when she comes into the session while feelings of anger or fear (usually in relation to Luisa) are still "live" and accessible. It is then that I can contain and hold her contradictory self-states in such a way that she can recognize and address both; my authentic and benign presence at these times is crucial, as is my ability to be gently playful. At the same time that I use these moments to make sense of and often reframe Cynthia's intense affects, I also use them to mentalize Luisa's intentions and mental states, often misread by her mother (Slade, in press). The following session, which occurred 1 year into the treatment, illustrates these points in a variety of ways. During the hour I worked on a number of levels to neutralize distorted representations of her child, increase Cynthia's own mentalizing capacities, and create a structure for unmetabolized and disruptive affects. In essence, by containing her rage and unpacking her projections, I helped Cynthia to provide more of an authentically secure base to Luisa, and helped her acknowledge feelings that belonged to her and not her daughter.

I came down to the waiting room to get Cynthia for our regularly scheduled 9:00 A.M. hour and saw that she had brought Luisa with her. Luisa looked shell-shocked, and a very worried look passed over her face when I came into the waiting room. She probably figured that soon she would be called upstairs, too. Cynthia came into my office and proceeded to tell me about an awful night they'd had. They had gone to the video store and chosen a movie to watch together before bed. While Cynthia had agreed to this plan, she had kept Luisa (who during this time did her usual fidgeting, etc.) waiting until nearly 11:00 P.M., when she finally agreed to sit down with her to watch the movie. Of course it was by then well past Luisa's bedtime. At midnight, Cynthia announced that it was too late to watch any more of the movie, and that Luisa had to go to bed. They paused the movie midstream. Luisa was of course wide awake and revved up at this point, and protested mightily. Cynthia insisted, and went to bed herself. She awoke at 2:00, and found Luisa awake in her own bedroom, doing her usual "odd" and furtive things. Cynthia erupted in a full rage, threatening and berating. She then sat down and watched the end of the movie by herself, with Luisa banished to her bedroom. She announced that the movie was going back the next day, and Luisa would not be allowed to see the end of it. Neither mother nor child slept much at all.

Cynthia felt indignant and vindicated. She so often described Luisa's badness, and here was hard evidence. This afternoon they were going to see Dr. Jenkins and tell her exactly what had happened. But I surprised her and surprised myself. With a smile, I gently teased her: "So, what terrible thing did she do this time?" (Translation: And exactly *why* did you get so angry?) To my relief, she paused and smiled, looking a little admonished, but also as if she was coming to her senses. In that instant she began to back down from her fury, and took a few steps back and considered that there might be another way to think about what had happened. Her fury had erupted when she had found Luisa still awake and mousing around at 2:00 A.M.; after all, she'd promised to go to bed, had violated their agreement by not going to sleep, and so on. "Kind of sounds like ADD boy kind of stuff to me," I said mildly, thinking of boys who take apart clocks, borrow and lose things, and so forth. I was also thinking about children who have trouble down-regulating after they've been excited.

She exhaled and paused. "You're right," she said, easing up a bit. By the end of the session, she realized that it was *she* who had delayed sitting down to watch the movie until 11:00 P.M. Luisa had repeatedly asked to start the movie, but Cynthia had continued to put it off in a way that in retrospect seemed to her rejecting. She recognized that she had ignored Luisa's wishes to have some time together and then had abruptly ended their pleasurable time together, sending Luisa into her "usual" mode of defense. I suggested that Luisa's behavior wasn't (at least consciously) malevolent, intentional, or bad; rather, it was her way of coping. She was then able to talk about how Luisa's behavior made her feel like a failure and like a bad mother; it also made her feel paranoid, as if Luisa was always doing things behind Cynthia's back.

"What do I do now?" she asked at the end of the session, both relieved and chagrined.

"You go downstairs and apologize, first of all, and then you two are going to go home and watch the end of the movie."

"And what do I tell Dr. Jenkins?"

"Nothing," I said, "it's Luisa's session." In essence, I guided her toward making reparation, something that no one in her own family of origin had ever done with her, but that she was now beginning to be able to do with Luisa.

Linking these rages and their obverse, fear and humiliation, to her childhood experience was more complicated for Cynthia, for dissociation and numbing had become well-worn defenses to protect her against painful memories and sensations. But over the course of the second year of our work together, Cynthia slowly became able to recognize the extent to which her rage and frightening behavior with Luisa could be understood as a reaction to her own childhood traumas, experiences she is less and less inclined to dissociate. As an example, she began a session some 2 months after the one reported above by talking about Emma's coming home from college, and how chaotic things had been. This followed an earlier discussion of how deeply dysregulated she is by the chaos when both kids are home and things feel out of control. She then very genuinely confessed that she had not wanted to come in, because she had lost it with Luisa immediately after our last session and hated to tell me. She had gone to a meeting near her home and had arranged that Luisa would pick her up after the meeting, with their dog. But Luisa never showed. Cynthia finally stalked home, and found her immersed in something on the computer. She reminded herself that because of her ADHD, Luisa can lose track of time and get totally absorbed in things. Nevertheless, she erupted in a rage—"One of the worst ever," she said miserably. She threatened to send Luisa to live with her father and (wicked) stepmother and berated her daughter for letting her down, not following through on her promises, and so on. She couldn't stop herself, even though Luisa at one point said to her, "You know, Mom, I think that this is about more than my not showing up with the dog. I think there's something else going on with you."

She calmed down enough to apologize to Luisa before bed, but was still very angry. They continued talking about it over the next few days. Cynthia felt worse and worse about it and repeatedly tried to reassure Luisa that she was terribly sorry. She described tucking her daughter into bed the next night and cradling Luisa's face in her hands. "I love you," she told Luisa. "This is the real deal, this is how I really feel . . . not that rage the other night. You're a great kid." I had the sense that she was trying, both for herself and Luisa, to differentiate between her sometimes hollow displays of affection and this, the real deal. She desperately wanted Luisa to believe that *this* was her authentic emotion.

She then started to spontaneously reflect on what had caused her to lose it. "I think it's my perfectionism . . . I always pressure myself to be perfect . . . perfect wife, house, children, et cetera." It felt to me like she was heading into a dissociated mode, and so I spoke. She had mentalized spontaneously while talking about very intense feelings of both anger and shame, but then had started to dissociate. I felt it needed to be kept live, and I felt it was crucial to link her response to Luisa to her own past. I interrupted her gently and said that I thought the perfectionism was a symptom. I said, "The real issue is trauma. You have to make sure everything is perfect so you can forestall the attack. You lived with such violence and chaos, you never knew when and what was coming next, the hitting, screaming, everything. Things are getting chaotic . . . your older daughter is coming home, you're going away [she added, "the dog is sick!"], things are starting to get overwhelming, and this terrifies you, because you don't know what is going to happen."

I was very specific, and she was right there with me. "As I'm listening to you, I'm thinking about Friday nights," she said, and then described her father coming home on Friday nights after being away for the week. Her mother would warn the children on Wednesday night that their father was coming home on Friday, and, as she put it, "from that moment on—we would all be wondering what would happen when he arrived. He would come in, put down his briefcase and his Gucci bag, juiced up from drinking on his first-class flight home, and we would never know—sometimes he would be fine, and sometimes he would fool us, he'd be in a good mood, but by midnight he'd be beating the shit out of my mom, or screaming at her or cornering her somewhere." Her language was direct, vivid, authentic, and absolutely coherent.

I got Cynthia off "remote" by specifically imagining what it was like for her to be a terrified, overwhelmed child. I used specific language and I tried to use imagery that I thought would evoke memories of her childhood. I don't think she would have had those associations if I had waited for them to emerge on their own. I think I needed to stimulate a visceral reaction in some way. I was helped, of course, by the fact that her negative affects were very live for her at that moment, having described the fight with her daughter in such graphic detail.

After she had described her father's returns in vivid detail, I gently said: "But this isn't Friday night." "I know," she agreed sadly. She then described with great clarity how she had several days earlier begun to feel overwhelmed by all that was "about to happen" with her children. There were so many details—things to do, and to work out. She briefly mentioned a conversation with her older daughter, which had made her feel ashamed and guilty, a very vulnerable state for her. I then said, "You know, having kids around can be like having little grenades explode. Usually they don't really hurt you, but if you're vulnerable to chaos and to anger, they feel like Friday night. It can feel very disorganizing." To which she replied, "It IS!"

With sadness, she then talked about seeing a resurgence of anxiety in Luisa, who was acting nervous, placating, apologetic, "insecure." She spontaneously said that she realizes that she is actually making Luisa feel the way she felt on Friday nights, and she doesn't want to do that. "I'm acting like my father . . . It's like I have this 'out of body' experience of becoming so enraged, and a part of me is standing there saying, 'Stop! Don't do this!' " With great feeling, she lamented the rages that take her over and sweep her away, and the damage she does to her daughter each time she erupts.

This session marked a huge step forward, because Cynthia used her understanding of her dysregulation in the present moment to reflect on the past. She was then able to use this understanding of the past to make sense of moments of extreme anger in relation to her daughter. Cynthia's danger points are the moments when she feels dysregulated and chaotic, or when she feels like a bad mother, *just like her own mother*. It is at these moments that—fearing the worst, and unable to turn to anyone to regulate or settle her, for her mother was also both frightened and frightening—she lashes out in desperate anger. I think what I did in the moment when I raised the issue of trauma was reframe her dysregulation and rage in a way to make it comprehensible and less shameful. She suddenly started to make sense to herself, and sense of the "out of body" experience of her anger. My port of entry was her dysregulation and high-intensity affect.

Often, shifts in the countertransference provided vital cues to where I needed to work. Early on, I frequently felt dysregulated and overwhelmed by Cynthia, whose humiliation at having been referred to me likely generated a great deal of internal upheaval. But as she settled in and started to trust me and our work, I was more often aware of becoming bored and restless as she shifted into "remote." My feelings of deadness became clues that something important was going on. Cynthia has the potential to be highly vulnerable within the transference, and for this reason I need to be especially careful to protect her and avoid any potential humiliation. While I expect Cynthia to bring the helpless–hostile dichotomy more directly into the transferential relationship at some point, she now needs to see and experience me primarily as an unambivalently held secure base. When the relationship feels too risky, she shifts into "remote." This is often the starting point in a session, after which I begin the slow work of reminding her that I am not going to hurt or frighten her.

Needless to say, these helpless–hostile "transferences"—or what Lyons-Ruth (Lyons-Ruth et al., 1999) would call "relational diatheses"— play themselves out in different ways in Cynthia's real-life relationships. Clearly, she is the aggressor in her relationship with Luisa; by contrast, she is far more placating and submissive in her romantic relationships, in her relationship to Emma, and in her relationship with her mother, who continues to find ways to shame and humiliate her to this day. Unfortunately for Luisa, who has functioned as a lightning rod for numerous unresolved traumas (the failed pregnancy and ensuing infertility, Cynthia's failed marriage and tormented affair), she is the one who most directly experiences her mother's rage, and who—as she gets older and more entrenched in the disorganized conundrum herself—is beginning to take it on as part of her own persona as well. Both sides of Cynthia's split internal world exist in all of her relationships, but each relationship is distinct in the degree to which one pole or the other defines its essential aspects.

CONCLUDING REMARKS

Thinking about Cynthia as *disorganized in relation to attachment* provides a crucial organizing structure for my work with her. First of all, it helps me imagine what it is like to be her, caught between being frightened and frightening, feeling helpless and hostile in relation to those she must care for or seek care from. I have the behavioral patterns as well as the representational patterns in mind when I work with her. Even more important, perhaps, I understand these patterns of ways of seeking care, or of coping with the absence of care in the face of danger and dysregulation. She makes sense to me in a particular way and I am thus able to help her make sense of herself. I see much of what she does as geared toward managing her fear and shame and short-circuiting her rage, well-established defenses that arose out of a childhood filled with violence, unpredictability, and chaos. The threatening mother and disrupted baby I described earlier capture many aspects of what I imagine Cynthia's experience to have been, namely the experience of being violated, being frightened, trying to keep up a good front, trying very hard not to get mad back. But as an adult she is also that angry mother (and, in her case even more, angry father), poking, assaulting, looming, her baby's fear invisible to her. Thus, the metaphors I use in my work with her are experience near and "fit" with her experience.

Fred Pine, one of my early and most significant mentors, described the impact of his work studying the separation–individuation process (Mahler, Pine, & Bergman, 1975) in a similar way:

> Early developmental research affects the practice of psychoanalysis in the language that the analyst (at times) uses in speaking to the patient, or more precisely, in the phenomena to which that language refers. Knowing the significance of early gaze and vocal/nonverbal interaction between mother and infant, aware of phenomena like the "practicing" of motor-independent activities, of shadowing, low-keyedness, and coercion—all drawn from Mahler's work—and feeling convinced of the power of early infant–mother bonding and the gap left when early attachment has been interrupted or underdeveloped, the analyst can at times speak to the patient in a language close to his or her early experience, hence more evocatively in terms of the recovering of memories and more empathically in terms of understanding inner experience . . . the other side of this coin is that the analyst can be attuned to certain behaviors of the patient that hark back to these early phenomena and thus can get cues to where the patient is at . . . For a language close to the patient's concrete experience is evocative in the way that visual images in a dream are suggestive for associative content, in the way that return to the site of an old experience leads to a rich recall of the past, in the way that the taste of a Madeleine released a flood of childhood memories in Marcel Proust. (1985, pp. 22–23)

Pine was describing how his work as a researcher had transformed his work with his adult patients. It had subtly changed the images in his own mind, changed the kinds of phenomena he noticed in patients' speech and behavior, and it had changed the kinds of things he said to patients. The more we know about childhood, he suggested, the richer our capacity to imagine our patients' experience, at multiple levels. After 25 years of immersion in attachment theory and research, I find that Pine's words capture exactly what it has meant to me to have attachment processes in mind when I work with adult patients. It doesn't supplant dynamic thinking, or erase all my years of experience in psychoanalytic supervision and psychoanalysis, but it has expanded what I hear and what I listen for. Put simply, I think that understanding the nature and function of attachment processes—as they are reflected in an adult's language, mentation, and behavior—allows me to *keep the child in mind in adult psychotherapy*, that is, to imagine my adult patient as a child, in moments of engagement with her primary objects. This understanding often helps me make sense of how she regulates affect, particularly in moments of high-intensity arousal. Most important, it often helps me find a way to speak to my patient and to her experience.

It is my experience with Cynthia that there is something hugely comforting about making sense of these moments in light of what Cynthia experienced and what she expects. I think my seeing Cynthia this way helps her. I think it helps her feel understood and held in mind in a nonjudgmental way. She does not like confessing to me, but she does not fear it. Because I inherently see her rages as comprehensible, and because I can put into words some of the reasons she does what she does, I am regulating to her. For the most part, she does not frighten me, nor does she make me angry. I appreciate her great courage and honesty, and I marvel at what she is willing to tackle in a relatively young treatment.

Thinking in terms of attachment organization also helps me understand and mentalize some of what Cynthia's own child may be experiencing. Because Cynthia is so avoidant of her own needs for comfort and safety, as they leave her vulnerable to fear and humiliation, she often misses Luisa's cues and fails to see her as a separate person with needs and feelings of her own (Slade, 2005). By giving voice to Luisa's internal experience I am working not only on repairing the splits *within* Cynthia, but within her relationships as well. She is slowly becoming a more authentic and reflective parent. This "ancillary" but crucial effect of individual psychotherapeutic work with adults who also happen to be parents is often overlooked in writings on adult psychotherapy and psychoanalysis. But changes in real relationships are as healing and transforming as changes in internal ones.

As I described above, crucial aspects of our work take place in moments of high-intensity arousal (see too Stern, 2004), moments that will reveal and hold the potential for transforming what I earlier termed the relational drama around careseeking. For Cynthia, careseeking was potentially terrifying and humiliating, both because of her parents' propensity to terrorize and shame, as well as the fact of her father's unpredictability and penchant for violence. Thus, moments in which she is both terrorized and terrorizing are ripe moments for reflection, mentalization, and change.

In this chapter I have used the data of my work with one adult psychotherapy case to illuminate some of the ways that thinking about attachment organization has affected my clinical work. This is consistent with my belief that case material provides the most immediate way of revealing these complex and subtle influences. But even case material cannot quite capture the ephemeral nature of influence and transformation. There is no way to specify precisely how my work as a psychoanalytic psychologist has been changed by my immersion in attachment theory and research. "How," as W. B. Yeats asked, in his poem "Among School Children" (1921/1996), "can we separate the dancer from the dance?"

ACKNOWLEDGMENTS

This chapter evolved from a presentation made to the Institute for Contemporary Psychoanalysis in Los Angeles on June 11, 2005. I am grateful to Helen Ziskind for asking me to write a paper I didn't think I had in me, and to Helen Grebow for setting the whole process in motion. I am also grateful to the Bridging the Gap Working Group, for once again providing a secure base for my explorations.

REFERENCES

Ainsworth, M. D. S., Blehar, M. C., Waters, E., & Wall, S. (1978). *Patterns of attachment: Psychological study of the Strange Situation.* Hillsdale, NJ: Erlbaum.

Barkley, R. A. (1997). *ADHD and the nature of self-control.* New York: Guilford Press.

Bowlby, J. (1969). *Attachment and loss: Vol. 1. Attachment.* New York: Basic Books.

Bowlby, J. (1973). *Attachment and loss: Vol. 2. Separation: Anxiety and anger.* New York: Basic Books.

Bowlby, J. (1980). *Attachment and loss: Vol. 3. Loss.* New York: Basic Books.

Bowlby, J. (1988). *A secure base: Parent–child attachment and healthy human development.* New York: Basic Books.

Brazelton, T. B., & Cramer, B. (1990). *The earliest relationship: parents, infants and the drama of early attachment.* Reading, MA: Addison-Wesley.

Fairbairn, W. R. D. (1952). *Psychoanalytic studies of the personality.* London: Routledge, Kegan, & Paul.

Fonagy, P. (2000). Attachment and borderline personality disorder. *Journal of the American Psychoanalytic Association, 48,* 1129–1146.

Fonagy, P. (2001). *Attachment theory and psychoanalysis.* New York: Other Press.

Fonagy, P., Gergely, G., Jurist, E., & Target, M. (2002). *Affect regulation, mentalization, and the development of the self.* New York: Other Press.

Fonagy, P., Steele, M., Steele, H., Leigh, T., Kennedy, R., Mattoon, G., et al. (1995). Attachment, the reflective self, and borderline states: The predictive specificity of the Adult Attachment Interview and pathological emotional development. In S. Goldberg, R. Muir, & J. Kerr (Eds.), *Attachment theory:*

Social, developmental and clinical perspectives (pp. 223–279). Hillsdale, NJ: Analytic Press.

Fonagy, P., & Target, M. (1996). Playing with reality: I. Theory of mind and the normal development of psychic reality. *International Journal of Psychoanalysis, 77,* 217–233.

Fonagy, P., & Target, M. (1998). Mentalization and the changing aims of child psychoanalysis. *Psychoanalytic Dialogues, 8,* 87–114.

Fraiberg, S. (1980). (Ed.). *Clinical studies in infant mental health.* New York: Harper & Row.

George, C., & Solomon, J. (1998, July). *Attachment disorganization at age six: Differences in doll play between punitive and caregiving children.* Paper presented at the meeting of the International Society for the Study of Behavioral Development, Bern, Switzerland.

Hesse, E., & Main, M. (2000). Disorganized infant, child, and adult attachment. *Journal of the American Psychoanalytic Association, 48,* 1097–1129.

Holmes, J. (1995). Something there is that doesn't love a wall: John Bowlby, attachment theory and psychoanalysis. In S. Goldberg, R. Muir, & J. Kerr (Eds.), *Attachment theory: Social, developmental and clinical perspectives* (pp. 19–45). Hillsdale, NJ: Analytic Press.

Lyons-Ruth, K., Bronfman, L., & Atwood, G. (1999). A relational diathesis model of hostile–helpless states of mind: Expressions in mother–infant interaction. In J. Solomon & C. C. George (Eds.), *Attachment disorganization* (pp. 33–70). New York: Guilford Press.

Lyons-Ruth, K., & Jacobvitz, D. (1999). Attachment disorganization: Unresolved loss, relational violence, and lapses in behavioral and attentional strategies. In J. Cassidy & P. R. Shaver (Eds.), *The handbook of attachment: Theory, research, and clinical applications* (pp. 520–554). New York: Guilford Press.

Mahler, M., Pine, F., & Bergman, A. (1975). *The psychological birth of the human infant.* New York: Basic Books.

Main, M. (1991). Metacognitive knowledge, metacognitive monitoring, and singular (coherent) vs. multiple (incoherent) model of attachment: Findings and directions for future research. In C. Parkes, J. Stevenson-Hinde, & P. Marris (Eds.), *Attachment across the life cycle* (pp. 127–160). London: Routledge.

Main, M. (1995). Recent studies in attachment: Overview, with selected implications for clinical work. In S. Goldberg, R. Muir, & J. Kerr (Eds.), *Attachment theory: Social, developmental and clinical perspectives* (pp. 407–475). Hillsdale, NJ: Analytic Press.

Main, M., & Hesse, E. (1990). Lack of mourning in adulthood and its relationship to infant disorganization: Some speculations regarding causal mechanisms. In M. Greenberg, D. Cicchetti, & M. Cummings (Eds.), *Attachment in the preschool years: Theory, research, and intervention* (pp. 161–182). Chicago: University of Chicago Press.

Main, M., Kaplan, N., & Cassidy, J. (1985). Security in infancy, childhood and adulthood: A move to the level of representation. In I. Bretherton & E. Waters (Eds.), Growing points in attachment theory and research. *Monographs of the Society for Research in Child Development, 50*(1–2, Serial No. 209), 66–104.

Mitchell, S. (1999). Attachment theory and the psychoanalytic tradition. *Psychoanalytic Dialogues, 9*, 85–108.

Pine, F. (1985). *Developmental theory and clinical process.* New Haven, CT: Yale University Press.

Slade, A. (1999a). Attachment theory and research: Implications for the theory and practice of individual psychotherapy with adults. In J. Cassidy & P. R. Shaver (Eds.), *Handbook of attachment: Theory, research and clinical applications* (pp. 575–594). New York: Guilford Press.

Slade, A. (1999b). Representation, symbolization and affect regulation in the concomitant treatment of a mother and child: Attachment theory and child psychotherapy. *Psychoanalytic Inquiry, 19*, 797–830.

Slade, A. (2000). The development and organization of attachment: Implications for psychoanalysis. *Journal of the American Psychoanalytic Association, 48*, 1147–1174.

Slade, A. (2004a). The move from categories to phenomena: Attachment processes and clinical evaluation. *Infant Mental Health Journal, 25*, 1–15.

Slade, A. (2004b). Two therapies: Attachment organization and the clinical process. In L. Atkinson & S. Goldberg (Eds.), *Attachment issues in psychopathology and intervention* (pp. 181–206). Hillsdale, NJ: Erlbaum.

Slade, A. (2005). Parental reflective functioning: An introduction. *Attachment and Human Development, 7*, 269–281.

Slade, A. (in press). Working with parents in child psychotherapy: Engaging reflective capacities. *Psychoanalytic Inquiry.*

Slade, A., Sadler, L. S., de Dios-Kenn, C., Webb, D., Ezepchick, J., & Mayes, L. (2005). Minding the Baby: A reflective parenting program. *Psychoanalytic Study of the Child, 60*, 74–100.

Slade, A., Sadler, L. S., & Mayes, L. C. (2005). Minding the Baby: Enhancing parental reflective functioning in a nursing/mental health home visiting program. In L. J. Berlin, Y. Ziv, L. Amaya-Jackson, & M. Greenberg (Eds.), *Enhancing early attachments: Theory, research, intervention, and policy* (pp. 152–177). New York: Guilford Press.

Stern, D. N. (1985). *The interpersonal world of the infant.* New York: Basic Books.

Stern, D. N. (2004). *The present moment in psychotherapy and everyday life.* New York: Norton.

Tronick, E. Z., & Weinberg, M. K. (1997). Depressed mothers and infants: Failure to form dyadic states of consciousness. In L. Murray & P. J. Cooper (Eds.), *Postpartum depression and child development* (pp. 54–84). New York: Guilford Press.

Winnicott, D. W. (1965). *Maturational processes and the facilitating environment.* New York: International Universities Press.

Yeats, W. B. (1996). *The collected poems of W. B. Yeats* (rev. 2nd ed.) (W. B. Yeats & Richard J. Finneran, Eds.). New York: Scribner Paperback Poetry.

Index

AAI. *See* Adult Attachment Interview
Abandonment–depression, 192
Acceptance, in resolved parents, 116–117
Adolescent boys, 91
Adopted children (previously maltreated)
  attachment relationships with adoptive
    parents and, 58–59
  common histories of, 65
  intergenerational transmission of
    attachment and, 65–66
  need for attachment figures, 61
  negative affect and, 75–76
  overriding avoidance behavior in, 76,
    81–82, 83
Adoption
  challenges of, 63–64
  foster children and, 102
  by foster parents, 102, 103–104
  significance of, 65
Adoption Intervention Study
  background to, 64–66
  case presentation
    background information, 69–71
    co-construction task, 71–72
    feedback intervention, 72–74
  changes in parental attitudes linked to
    the co-construction task, 77–78
  changes in parental attitudes to the self
    and the child, 76–77
  co-construction assessment, 67–69
  discussion, 79–83
  key features of, 66
  methodology, 66–67
  reliability, 75–76
Adoptive parents
  attachment facilitating behavior and,
    80–81, 83
  attachment relationships with previ-
    ously maltreated children, 58–59
  changes in attitudes to the self and the
    child, 76–77
  co-construction task and, 71–72, 77–78
  feeling more attached to the child, 78
  feeling more competent, 78
  feeling the child to be more acceptable,
    77–78
  negative affect in adopted children and,
    75–76
  overriding avoidance behavior in
    adopted children, 76, 81–82, 83
Adult Attachment Interview (AAI), 167, 168
  assessing states of resolution with, 111
  significance of, 3–4, 64
Affect regulation, 188, 228
Aggression
  within the attachment relationship,
    158–159
  in insecure preschoolers, 207
Alien self, 231–232
Anger, in unresolved parents, 125–126

Anxiety, infants and, 231
Arousal regulation, 228
ASD. *See* Autism spectrum disorder
Attachment and Bio-behavioral Catch-up
    intervention, 104
Attachment/Attachment relationships
    careseeking and, 228–229
    co-construction task and, 78
    dyadic and triadic, 92–93
    effects of childhood trauma on, 139,
        166–167
    implicit relational knowing and, 176
    importance to previously maltreated,
        adopted children, 61
    influence the child's response to
        trauma, 139–140, 144–145
    intergenerational transmission in non-
        biological dyads, 65–66
    between maltreated children and adop-
        tive parents, 58–59
    relationship to commitment, 100–101
    using to facilitate recovery from trauma
        in children, 145–147
Attachment classifications, 227, 229
Attachment-deflecting behavior, overriding
    in adopted children, 76, 81–82, 83
Attachment-facilitating behavior
    adoptive parents and, 58–59, 83
    co-construction assessment, 67–69, 80–81
    See also Adoption Intervention Study
Attachment quality, 92
Attachment theory
    assumptions underlying, 63
    challenges of adoption, 63–64
    Circle of Security perspective on, 173–174
    concept of commitment and, 91–93
    historical review of, 62–64
    psychoanalysis and, 226
Autism spectrum disorder (ASD)
    parents resolved regarding the child's
        diagnosis, 114–121
    parents unresolved regarding the child's
        diagnosis, 121–128
Autonomous-secure state, 64
Avoidance behavior
    in adoptive parents, 83
    overriding in previously maltreated,
        adopted children, 76, 81–82, 83
    in traumatized children, 140

"Baby watchers," 60
Battered mothers, 142, 154

Birth parents, providing care to prior to
    separation from children, 103

Caregivers
    biological importance of, 90, 101
    commitment to children and, 90–91.
        See also Commitment
    and the consequences of domestic vio-
        lence for children, 141–142
Careseeking, 228–229
Child abuse, by battered mothers, 142
Child behavior
    avoidance, 140
    effects on commitment from caregivers,
        100
    in insecure attachments, 205
    maternal insightfulness and, 31, 33
    miscuing, 173
    parental resolution and, 130–131
Childhood trauma
    attachment relationships affect recovery
        from, 139–140, 145–147
    the attachment system influences
        response to, 144–145
    avoidance behavior and, 140
    denial and, 154
    domestic violence and, 141–143, 166
    impact on attachment relationships, 139
    therapeutic approach to. *See* Child–
        parent psychotherapy
    understanding from perspectives of
        attachment and trauma theories,
        140, 144, 166–167
Child–parent psychotherapy (CPP)
    assessing trauma and attachment–
        caregiving relationships, 146
    in a therapeutic preschool, 221–223
    attachment and trauma-focused goals
        of, 147, 166–168
    case presentation, 147–165
        attachment relationships in children,
            149, 150
        clinical case formulation, 152
        mother–child relationships, 151–152
        mother's attachment history, 150–151
        mother's trauma history and post-
            traumatic stress symptoms, 150
        traumatic stress symptoms in chil-
            dren, 148, 149–150
        treatment sessions, 152–165
    establishing safety, 155
    goals with parents, 151

outcomes, 165–166
premises of, 145, 166
speaking about domestic violence and, 154
termination of treatment, 163
trauma narratives and, 161
Children
experiences with disorganized attachments, 231–232
internal working models and, 204–205, 208
maternal insightfulness and, 31–32, 33, 34–35
"miscuing," 173
trauma and. See Childhood trauma
See also Adopted children; Child behavior; Foster children; Infants; Insecure children; Preschoolers
Children's Center, 35–36, 209–214. See also Therapeutic preschools
Circle of Security (COS) Project
case presentation, 179–200
concept of change in, 188
core sensitivities, 177–178
establishing change in parents, 185, 187
goals of, 176–177
intervention overview, 173–177
parent's views of the child's needs and, 187
purpose and focus of, 172–173
Circle of Security Interview (COSI), 103, 175, 179, 184
Co-construction assessment/task
attachment facilitating behaviors and, 68–69, 80–81
case presentation, 69–74
changes in parental attitudes related to, 77–78
coding, 68, 86–89
negative cyclical effect during, 80
overview of, 67–68
scoring strategies, 79–80
sharing filmed interactions with parents, 82
Cognitive distortions, in unresolved parents, 127
Commitment
associations with other variables, 99–101
attachment theory and, 91–93
examples of high and low levels in foster parents, 93–99
importance of, 101–102
relationship to attachment, 100–101
strategies for enhancing in foster care, 103–104

surrogate caregivers and, 90–91
Competence, parental, 78
Core sensitivities, 177–178, 184
COSI. See Circle of Security Interview
CPP. See Child–parent psychotherapy

Depression
abandonment–depression, 192
in unresolved parents, 126–127
Detachment, 149
Developmental disorders
parental resolution with regard to the child's diagnosis, 109–110
Disengaged mothers, 55–56
Disorganized adults, 127, 232
Disorganized attachment
aspects of disorganization in, 231–232
case presentations, 229–245
child identification with the parent's state of mind, 232
domestic violence as risk factor, 141–142
fear and, 230, 231
markers of, 234–236
psychotherapeutic approaches to, 245–248
symptoms in traumatized children, 143
trauma and, 166–167
unresolved parents and, 112
Disorganized–confused parents, 127. See also Disorganized adults
Disorganized/unresolved attachment, 227
Domestic violence
denial and, 154
impact on children, 140, 141–143, 166
impact on the attachment–caregiving system, 141–142
trauma occurs from witnessing, 142–143, 166
Dyadic attachment, 92, 93

Earned security, 196
Esteem sensitivity, 178

Family violence. See Domestic violence
Fear, disorganized attachment and, 230, 231
"Forty-Four Juvenile Thieves" (Bowlby), 91
Foster care, strategies for enhancing commitment in, 103–104
Foster care system
clinical implications of commitment studies, 102–104

Foster care systems *(cont.)*
numbers of children adopted and
awaiting adoption, 102
Foster children
with babies, providing support to, 103
factors affecting commitment to, 99–100
importance of caregiver commitment
to, 102
Foster parents
adopting children and, 102, 103–104
creating conditions that encourage
commitment to children, 103–104
high and low levels of commitment to
children, 91, 93–99
importance of commitment in
caregiving, 102
providing training and support to, 104
variables affecting commitment to children, 99–100

Holding environment, 210
Hypervigilance, 157–158

"Ideal grandmother" concept, 211–212
Implicit relational knowing, 176
Incoherence, in disorganized adults, 235
Infant–parent relationship
assessment, 5–28
parent's need for the child to be a certain way, 19, 21–22
prenatal perceptions of parents and, 10–11
Infants
anxiety and, 231
careseeking and, 228–229
experiences with disorganized attachments, 231–232
Insecure attachments, 112
avoidance behavior and, 140
Circle of Security intervention, 173–
177
consequences for preschoolers, 206–
208
dysfunctional behavior in children and,
205
treatment strategies for children, 205–206
Insecure children
deficits in caregiving and, 174
dysfunctional behavior and, 205
"miscuing," 173
See also Insecure attachments
Insecure/disorganized attachment, 112
Insecurity, types of, 64
Insight, 34

Insightfulness
attributes underlying the capacity for,
34–35
defined, 31, 33
disengaged mothers and, 55–56
effects of, 31–32, 56
importance of enhancing in parents,
32–33, 56
Insightfulness Assessment
case presentation (Anna and Tom)
posttreatment assessment, 42–46
pretreatment assessment, 36–42
case presentation (Doris and Debra)
posttreatment assessment, 50–54
pretreatment assessment, 46–50
classifications within, 34, 55
clinical implications of, 54–56
overview of, 33–36
Internal working models
in child development, 204
children's dysfunctional behavior and,
204–205
core sensitivities, 177–178
in insecure preschoolers, 208

Juvenile thieves, 91

Loss
adjustment to, 110–111, 113
attachment research on the resolution
of, 111–112
Bowlby's theory of, 110–111

Maltreated children. *See* Adopted children
(previously maltreated)
Minnesota Longitudinal Study, 119–200
Miscuing, 173
Mothers
battered, 142
disengaged, 55–56
insightfulness and. *See* Insightfulness
resolution and sensitivity, 130–131. *See
also* Resolution
traumatized, parenting and, 158
Mourning, 110–111
Music, Circle of Security intervention
and, 176

Narratives
Working Model of the Child Interview
and, 9
See also Trauma narratives
Negative affect, 75–76

Noninsightful/disengaged mothers, 55
Nurturing, 211

"On Knowing What You Are Not
    Supposed to Know" (Bowlby), 154
Oxytocin, 101

Parental competence, 78
Parental resolution. *See* Resolution
Parent–child interactions
    mismatches and, 60
    prelinguistic, 60–61
    research studies in, 60–61
Parent–child psychotherapy. *See* Child–
    parent psychotherapy
Parent–child relationship
    changes in caregiving behavior and,
        194–195
    parental resolution and, 129–131
Parenting, traumatized mothers and, 158
Parenting Stress Index (PSI), 67, 76, 77
Parents
    behavior is affected by resolution state,
        129–130, 131
    Circle of Security perspective on, 173–174
    core sensitivities, 177–178
    discussing feelings about the child's
        ASD diagnosis, 132–133
    disorganized–confused, 127
    feelings of competence, 78
    insightfulness and. *See* Insightfulness
    internal disorganization and, 232
    "miscuing" by insecure children, 173
    negative representations of the child,
        207, 208–209
    providing care to prior to separation
        from children, 103
    resolved, 114–121
    unresolved, 121–128
    under used capacity, 182
    See also Adoptive parents; Foster parents
Parent–therapist relationship, 188
Pervasive developmental disorder not
        otherwise specified (PDD NOS),
        114, 128
Play, developing trauma narratives and, 161
Posttraumatic stress disorder (PTSD)
    avoidance behavior and, 140
    caregivers impact resolution of symp-
        toms, 145
    in child witnesses of domestic violence,
        142–143
    diagnostic criteria in children, 143

Prelinguistic interactions, 60–61
Preschoolers
    consequences of insecure attachments
        for, 206–208
    negative parental representations and,
        207, 208–209
    See also Therapeutic preschools
Proximity, 206, 207
PSI. *See* Parenting Stress Index
Psychoanalysis, 226–227
PTSD. *See* Posttraumatic stress disorder

RDI. *See* Reaction to Diagnosis Interview
Reaction to Diagnosis Interview (RDI)
    coding, 133
    overview of, 113–114
    research findings from, 128–131
    using in clinical practice, 132–134
Reactive aggression, 207
Reflection, 188
Reflective functioning, 176–177
Relationship assessment model, 5–28. *See
    also* Working Model of the Child
    Interview
Relationship-based treatment
    in a therapeutic preschool, 209–214
    case presentation
    case formulation, 218–219
    child–parent psychotherapy, 221–223
    initial interview, 214–218
    summary, 223–224
    therapeutic preschool intervention,
        219–221
Relationship-diathesis model, 144–145
Reorganization, as the outcome of
        mourning, 110
Resolution
    acceptance and, 116–117
    changes in parental feelings, thoughts,
        and actions, 115–116
    the child's behavior and, 130–131
    consequences of the lack of, 111–112
    defined, 112–113
    importance of, 134–135
    of loss or trauma, 111–112
    maternal sensitivity and, 130
    parental behavior and, 129–130, 131
    raising awareness of among profession-
        als, 134
    with respect to the child's diagnosis,
        112–114
    resolved parents, 114–121
    unresolved parents, 121–128

Resolution *(cont.)*
 severity of the child's diagnosis and, 128–129
 significance of, 109–110
 subclassifications, 119–121
 suspending the search for reasons, 117–118
 time elapsed since the child's diagnosis and, 129
Resolved-action oriented parents, 120–121, 123
Resolved-feeling oriented parents, 119–120
Resolved parents
 acceptance, 116–117
 central features characterizing, 114–115
 changes in feelings, thoughts, and actions, 115–116
 subclassifications, 119–121
 suspending the search for reasons, 117–118
Resolved-thinking oriented parents, 119
Rhythmic coupling, 61
Role reversal, 181

Safety sensitivity, 178
Secure attachments
 child behavior and, 205
 expression of negative affects by children, 207
 normal development of, 206
Security, earned, 196
Self, alien, 231–232
Sensitivity, maternal resolution and, 130
Separation sensitivity, 178
"Shark Music," 176, 185, 188, 194
Social workers, in the Adoption Intervention Study, 67
SSP. *See* Strange Situation Procedure
Still-face episode, 7
Story Stem Assessment Profile, 67
Strange Situation Procedure (SSP), 92, 93, 141, 167, 168
 Circle of Security intervention and, 175, 179
Strengths and Difficulties Questionnaire, 67, 76, 77
Surrogate caregivers, 90–91. *See also* Foster parents

Tavistock Clinic, 62
Therapeutic preschools
 case presentation, 214–224
 relationship-based treatment in, 209–214

This Is My Baby (TIMB) interview
 commitment ratings, 107–108
 examples of commitment levels, 94–98
 interrater reliability, 99
 interview questions, 107
 overview of, 94
 social desirability biases and, 98–99
 validity, 99
TIMB. *See* This Is My Baby Interview
"Time-In Parenting," 190, 222
Trauma
 attachment research on the resolution of, 111–112
 See also Childhood trauma
Trauma narratives, 161–163
Traumatized mothers, parenting and, 158
"Triad," 192
Triadic attachment, 92, 93

Unresolved–angry preoccupation parents, 125–126
Unresolved–depressed parents, 126–127
Unresolved–emotionally overwhelmed parents, 123–125
Unresolved–neutralizing parents, 122–123
Unresolved parents
 characteristic features of, 121–122, 131
 disorganized attachment and, 112
 subclassifications, 122–128
 the working model of the child and, 131
"Unthought known," 183

WMCI. *See* Working Model of the Child Interview
Working Model of the Child Interview (WMCI)
 case presentation
  clinician's summing up with the mother, 26–28
  initial referral, 6–7
  interactional assessment, 7
  interview excerpts, 7–25
  introduction to, 5–6
  mother's representation of the infant, 25
  preliminary formulation, 25–26
  treatment summary, 28
 initial probes, 9
 narrative and, 9
 overview of, 4, 28
 validation of, 4